Concise Handbook of Epidemiology
(Second Edition)

Authored by

Jalal-Eddeen Abubakar Saleh
Field Presence Cluster
World Health Organization, Nigeria

Concise Handbook of Epidemiology (Second Edition)

Author: Jalal-Eddeen Abubakar Saleh

ISBN (Online): 978-981-5274-73-8

ISBN (Print): 978-981-5274-74-5

ISBN (Paperback): 978-981-5274-75-2

© 2024, Bentham Books imprint.

Published by Bentham Science Publishers Pte. Ltd. Singapore. All Rights Reserved.

First published in 2024.

need for a court order if at any point you breach any terms of this License Agreement. In no event will any delay or failure by Bentham Science Publishers in enforcing your compliance with this License Agreement constitute a waiver of any of its rights.

3. You acknowledge that you have read this License Agreement, and agree to be bound by its terms and conditions. To the extent that any other terms and conditions presented on any website of Bentham Science Publishers conflict with, or are inconsistent with, the terms and conditions set out in this License Agreement, you acknowledge that the terms and conditions set out in this License Agreement shall prevail.

Bentham Science Publishers Pte. Ltd.
80 Robinson Road #02-00
Singapore 068898
Singapore
Email: subscriptions@benthamscience.net

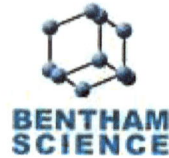

BENTHAM SCIENCE

CONTENTS

FOREWORD

It is with immense pleasure and anticipation that I introduce the second edition of the "Concise Handbook of Epidemiology." In the ever-evolving landscape of public health and disease prevention, this updated edition stands as a beacon of knowledge, guiding all who seek to comprehend the intricate science of epidemiology.

This comprehensive handbook navigates the entire spectrum of epidemiological inquiry, from foundational principles in Chapter 1 to the exploration of epidemiology in diverse local contexts in Chapter 9. It equips readers with the essential tools to understand and analyze epidemiological data, fostering a sense of responsibility and commitment to improving global health outcomes.

Chapter 1 lays the groundwork by introducing readers to the essence of epidemiological thought and practice, serving as the cornerstone for subsequent chapters. Chapter 2 delves into the heart of epidemiology, exploring essential models and frameworks that underpin our understanding of disease transmission. Chapter 3 acts as a compass, guiding readers through research design paradigms and statistical tools crucial for precise data analysis.

The vigilant eye of epidemiology is exemplified in Chapter 4, where readers explore disease surveillance systems and the art of outbreak detection and response through real-world case studies. Chapter 5 imparts the language fluency required for interpreting data with acumen, delving into foundational statistical concepts. Chapter 6 escorts readers to the frontiers of the discipline, unfolding advanced statistical techniques and addressing emerging challenges.

Chapter 7 showcases the practical dimensions of epidemiological principles, from influencing health policy to real-life case studies, engaging readers in active learning. Chapter 8 invites contemplation of the future of epidemiology, exploring innovations, ethical considerations, and the collective responsibility to shape the field's trajectory.

In a world of diverse regions and communities, Chapter 9 emphasizes the adaptability of epidemiological methods to local contexts, extolling the virtues of community engagement and narrating the stories of local epidemiology through case studies.

As readers embark on this journey, whether as students, researchers, healthcare professionals, or policymakers, I encourage embracing the wisdom within these pages. May this handbook serve as a constant source of guidance, inspiration, and enlightenment, empowering readers to contribute meaningfully to global community well-being.

I extend heartfelt gratitude to the author for crafting this invaluable resource and commend readers for their commitment to public health. With each turn of the page, we enhance our collective ability to address today's health challenges and forge a healthier, more resilient tomorrow.

Welcome to the realm of epidemiology – a convergence of science, compassion, and determination to safeguard and enhance the well-being of our communities.

Professor Zubairu Iliyasu
Bayero University, Kano, Nigeria

PREFACE

In the ever-evolving realm of public health and disease prevention, epidemiology stands as a sentinel, diligently observing, analysing, and deciphering the complex patterns of health and disease. The second edition of the "Concise Handbook of Epidemiology" comes with great pleasure and enthusiasm. Building upon the foundations I laid in the first edition, this updated volume embarks on a comprehensive journey through the multifaceted landscape of epidemiology, providing a concise yet robust guide for novice learners and seasoned practitioners.

Chapter 1: Foundations of Epidemiology In this opening chapter, I delve into the fundamental principles that underpin epidemiology. From understanding the nature of health and disease to exploring the various subfields within epidemiology, we lay the groundwork for a deeper exploration of this dynamic discipline.

Chapter 2: Epidemiological Models and Frameworks Chapter 2 introduces the reader to the epidemiological models and frameworks that are scaffolding for understanding disease transmission and progression. We unravel the intricacies of the epidemiologic triad, the chain of infection, and the natural history of the disease, providing the reader with essential tools to analyse health challenges.

Chapter 3: Epidemiological Research Design Research design is the compass that guides epidemiologists in their quest to uncover patterns and causality. Chapter 3 navigates through different research paradigms, study types, and the practical aspects of conducting epidemiological investigations. Statistical tools essential for data analysis are also explored.

Chapter 4: Disease Surveillance and Outbreak Investigations Disease surveillance is the guardian of public health, and in Chapter 4, I explore the mechanisms that underpin this essential function. Discover how outbreaks are detected, investigated, and controlled through insightful case studies and real-world examples.

Chapter 5: Statistical Methods Statistics is the language of epidemiology, and Chapter 5 equips the reader with the vocabulary and tools to interpret data effectively. From fundamental concepts to statistical inference and mathematical modelling, this chapter empowers readers with the skills needed for rigorous analysis.

Chapter 6: Advanced Epidemiological Methods As epidemiology continues to evolve, Chapter 6 guides readers through advanced statistical techniques and the impact of genomics on epidemiological research. It also addresses emerging challenges and opportunities that shape the future of the discipline.

Chapter 7: Applications and Case Studies Epidemiological knowledge comes to life through its application. Chapter 7 immerses readers in the practical aspects of epidemiological practice, from influencing health policy to real-life case studies that illustrate the principles in action. Exercises and questions challenge the reader's understanding.

Chapter 8: Future Directions and Challenges In Chapter 8, I peer into the future of epidemiology. Explore innovations in methods, grapple with ethical considerations, and join in shaping the trajectory of this ever-evolving field.

Chapter 9: Epidemiology in Local Context No two regions are the same, and Chapter 9 emphasises the importance of adapting epidemiological methods to local contexts. Learn how community engagement and case studies in local epidemiology can enhance the relevance and impact of the reader's work.

This handbook is not merely a compilation of facts and figures but an invitation to embark on a journey of discovery and empowerment. Whether the reader is a student, researcher, healthcare practitioner, or policymaker, the "Concise Handbook of Epidemiology" offers a valuable resource to enhance his understanding of the field. I encourage readers to engage with its contents, apply its principles, and contribute to advancing public health worldwide.

As readers turn the pages of this book, it is hoped that the knowledge within ignites their curiosity, inspires their passion for epidemiology, and equips them to make meaningful contributions to the health and well-being of our global community.

Thanks for embarking on this epidemiological journey with this revised edition. I hope this handbook serves as a valuable resource as readers navigate the dynamic and vital field of epidemiology. Together, we can address today's health challenges and shape a healthier future for all.

Disclaimer:

The views expressed in this book are mine and do not reflect the official position or policies of the WHO. Similarly, the content of this book ensured objectivity, avoided being impartial, and was not influenced by my affiliation with the WHO.

Jalal-Eddeen Abubakar Saleh
Field Presence Cluster
World Health Organization, Nigeria

DEDICATION

This book is dedicated to the pillars of my life (my dear parents, my loving wife, and my remarkable children) and the global community of epidemiologists who continue to shape our world.

CHAPTER 1

Foundations of Epidemiology

Abstract: This chapter lays the groundwork for understanding the principles, methods, and applications of epidemiology. Beginning with an introduction to the field, it delves into the intricacies of health and disease, exploring various epidemiological research fields and methodologies. The chapter elucidates the measurement of disease occurrence and highlights the significance, successes, and real-world applications of epidemiology.

Keywords: Epidemiology, Health, Disease, Research Methods, Disease Occurrence, Applications.

INTRODUCTION TO EPIDEMIOLOGY

The Role of Epidemiology in Public Health

Epidemiology serves as the cornerstone of public health, playing a pivotal role in understanding, monitoring, and improving the health of populations. It is the science that investigates the patterns, causes, and consequences of health and disease in communities, underscoring that clinical practice and health policy cannot be based on clinical experience alone but on scientific evidence as well. Epidemiologists help to assess the efficiency of health interventions, such as sanitary measures in controlling faeco-oral diseases, the effectiveness and efficiency of health services using specific parameters that include the duration of hospital stay for a particular condition, the impact of reducing unleaded petrol in lead poisoning, *etc*. It is critical to mention that a wide range of epidemiological methods are used for disease surveillance, outbreak investigations, hazards and risk factor assessment, and other health-related events [1 - 3].

Epidemiologists are like disease detectives, diligently examining data and evidence to identify health trends, risk factors, and opportunities for intervention. So, there is a need to highlight the significance of epidemiology in medical and public health practice and in the methods used to study health and disease. It is considered critical and a prerequisite to appraise the evidence obtained in the scientific literature, providing scientists with the necessary skills to provide evidence-based healthcare and clearly distinguish good from flawed science. Likewise, the results of epidemiological studies guide not only public health professionals but also other scientists, including health economists, health policy analysts, and health services managers [1 - 3].

Epidemiology offers several critical functions in public health:

1.Disease Surveillance: Epidemiologists monitor the occurrence of diseases and health events, tracking outbreaks, and ensuring timely responses to emerging threats.

2.Identifying Risk Factors: By conducting rigorous research, epidemiologists uncover the factors that contribute to the development of diseases, from lifestyle choices to environmental exposures.

3.Evaluating Interventions: Public health programs and policies are assessed for their effectiveness through epidemiological studies, ensuring resources are directed where they are most needed.

4.Shaping Health Policy: Epidemiological evidence guides policymakers in making informed decisions, from setting priorities to allocating resources for healthcare and prevention.

5.Preventing and Controlling Disease: Epidemiologists develop strategies for disease prevention and control, whether through vaccination campaigns, health education, or environmental interventions.

Historical Evolution and Milestones

The roots of epidemiological thinking can be traced back to ancient civilizations, but modern epidemiology has evolved significantly over the centuries. Epidemiological thinking started nearly 2,500 years ago, in 400 BC, when Hippocrates, often regarded as the father of medicine, observed that environmental factors influence disease occurrence. His work laid the foundation for the rational study of disease causation. In his early writings on 'Airs, Waters and Places,' Hippocrates explained disease occurrence using a rational approach and suggested that the development of human disease might be related to an individual's external and personal environment [4 - 6].

In 1662, the analysis of mortality data by John Graunt in London marked a turning point in epidemiology. He made a remarkable contribution to epidemiology when he published analysed mortality data which quantified the patterns of birth, death, and disease occurrence, pointing out disparities between males and females, high infant mortality, differences between urban and rural settings, and seasonal variations [4 - 6].

In 1800, William Farr, regarded as the father of modern vital statistics and surveillance, systematically collected vital statistics. He evaluated, analysed, and reported vital statistics to the responsible health authorities and the general public. The work by Farr led to the development of essential practices in today's vital statistics and disease classification [6, 7].

In 1854, John Snow, an anaesthesiologist considered the "father of field epidemiology," conducted a series of investigations in London to unravel the mystery behind the Golden Square of London cholera epidemic. His investigation, which was twenty years before the advent of the microscope, used classical descriptive epidemiology to unravel the mystery. During the cholera outbreak, Snow believed water to be the source of the infection. He generated and tested a hypothesis using analytical epidemiology. Through the use of 'dots and maps', he investigated the cholera epidemic by determining the locations of people with the disease and the water pump that served them (Table **1**) [8].

Table 1. Deaths from cholera in the districts of London supplied by Southwark and Lambeth companies (8th July - 26th August 1854) [8].

Company Name	Populations (1851)	Cholera Deaths (n)	Cholera Death Rate (per 1000 population)
Southwark	167654	844	5.0
Lambeth	19133	18	0.9

Snow, taking the biological, chemical, physical, sociological, and political processes into consideration, highlighted the clustering of cases on his spot map; his report showed that most of the cases were people who got their water supply from pump A (the Broad Street pump) as against those whose source of water supply was either pump B or C [4 - 6]. Similarly, using the 1854 London cholera outbreak data, Snow reported that the districts with the highest death rates had their water supply from the Lambeth Company and the Southwark and Vauxhall Company. These two companies got their water from the Thames River, whose intake points were downstream from London, which had the likelihood of getting contaminated by London sewage discharged into it. The outcome of the research conducted by Snow impacted public health policy as it resulted in improvements in the water supply system. However, despite the advancement in epidemiology, cholera outbreaks are still prevalent in developing countries, especially among poor populations, and often with fatal outcomes [9].

Epidemiology recorded significant successes in the late 19th and early 20th centuries in applying epidemiological methods to investigate disease occurrence; initially, the focus was on acute infectious diseases, but later, it included chronic non-communicable diseases (NCDs) around the mid-20th century. The focus of the NCDs was to look at the causal association between a disease and exposure (*e.g.*, smoking and lung cancer, and cholesterol and cardiovascular diseases) [10, 11]. Similarly, applied epidemiology was extended to cover other related fields, such as injury and molecular genetics, to explore specific pathways and have a clearer picture of the influencers or risks of developing certain diseases [12, 13].

However, despite the advances recorded in the discipline, epidemiologists continue to face increasing challenges in the form of biological warfare and bioterrorism, emerging and reemerging infectious agents, such as the Ebola Virus, Human Immunodeficiency Virus (HIV), Middle East Respiratory Syndrome (MERS), severe acute respiratory syndrome (SARS), Avian Influenza, Multi-drug Resistant Mycobacterium Tuberculosis (MDR-TB), and the COVID-19 pandemic in late 2019 [14 - 18].

Exercise 1: Reflecting on Local Epidemiological Milestones

This exercise encourages readers to connect the principles of epidemiology to their specific local context, fostering a deeper understanding of its relevance and significance in addressing local health issues.

   i. Now, let us apply these concepts to your local context. Consider the following questions:
  ii. Are there any notable disease outbreaks or health events that have shaped public health in your region or community?
 iii. What were the key milestones or discoveries in the history of epidemiology that have had a direct impact on the health of your local population?
  iv. How have local epidemiologists and public health professionals contributed to addressing health challenges unique to your region?
   v. What are the current public health priorities and challenges in your community, and how can epidemiological approaches be used to address them effectively?

Exercise 2: Defining Health Challenges in Your Region

This exercise empowers readers to apply epidemiological concepts to their local context, fostering a deeper understanding of the health challenges specific to their region and encouraging critical thinking about potential solutions.

i. To apply these concepts to your local context, consider the following exercise:
ii. Identify Local Health Challenges: Research and document the current health challenges and trends in your region or community. These challenges can include infectious diseases, non-communicable diseases, environmental health issues, or social determinants affecting health.
iii. Define the Scope: For each identified health challenge, define its scope by quantifying the incidence, prevalence, and affected populations. If available, gather data and statistics to support your analysis.
iv. Identify Risk and Protective Factors: Explore the risk factors contributing to these health challenges, such as lifestyle behaviors, environmental exposures, or socioeconomic factors. Moreover, identify any protective factors that may mitigate the risks.
v. Examine Local Definitions of Health: Investigate how health and disease are perceived and defined within your community. Are there cultural or societal factors that influence these definitions?
vi. Propose Interventions: Based on your analysis, propose interventions and strategies to address these health challenges effectively. Consider preventive measures, health promotion campaigns, or policy changes.

UNDERSTANDING HEALTH AND DISEASE

Definition and Scope

Defining health and disease is fundamental to the practice of epidemiology. These definitions serve as the building blocks upon which epidemiologists assess and address public health issues.

Health is a multifaceted concept encompassing physical, mental, and social well-being. The World Health Organization (WHO) defines health as "a state of complete physical, mental, and social well-being and not merely the absence of disease or infirmity." This holistic perspective emphasizes that health extends beyond the absence of illness to include overall well-being [19].

Disease refers to an abnormal condition or disorder that impairs the normal functioning of the body or mind. Diseases can be acute (short-term) or chronic (long-term), infectious or non-infectious, and they may manifest in various forms, from physical symptoms to mental health challenges [19].

The term epidemiology, derived from Greek, means **epi** 'upon', **demos'** people', and **logy** 'study'. It could be defined as a study that deals with the ***distribution*** and ***determinants*** of ***health events*** in a specified population for appropriate public health actions (*i.e.*, to prevent and control health problems) [16 - 18].

With disease surveillance at the centre of it all and considered the foundation of epidemiology, the study of diseases could be either through observational or experimental research.

The discipline of epidemiology is unique because it provides an approach for public health professionals to clearly understand **health and disease** and the **forces or factors** that influence them. It also enables public health professionals to study diseases and assess the **effectiveness of health care services** and the **impact of health care interventions**. The information obtained at the end is then used to prevent disease, protect and promote good health, and conduct clinical and health services research [16, 17].

Although various methods are used in epidemiological investigations, the most common is through **surveillance and descriptive studies** to look at disease distribution – the 'who, when, and where' and **analytical studies** – the 'how and why' to help understand the disease determinants. This approach would help to institute preventive and control measures that promote, protect, and restore the health of individuals or groups.

Therefore, it is pertinent to understand the three keywords mentioned in the epidemiology definition – **distribution**, **determinants**, and **health events** [4 - 6].

1. Distribution refers to the frequency and pattern of health events. The frequency, which is measured by the rates and risk of health events, requires the number of occurrences of the event within a given population and at a given time. In contrast, the pattern refers to the occurrence of health-related events by time (seasonal, annual, daily, weekly, *etc.*), place (geographical, urban/rural setting, workplace or school, *etc.*), and people (age, gender, marital status, SES, social behaviours, *etc.*). Distribution describes the 'who, when, and where' health-related events occur.

2. Determinants refer to the factors that influence health-related events, such as risk factors or protective factors; these include biological, chemical, physical, social, cultural, economic, genetic, and behavioural changes. As assumed by epidemiologists, disease occurrence in a population is only possible when risk factors or determinants come into existence. Epidemiologists search for these determinants, using an analytical approach to the cause and answer the "Why" and "How" of such events. To answer these, epidemiologists look at the risk factors that assess the genetic composition of individuals, their demographic characteristics, social behaviours, and any possible environmental exposure to prompt public health measures.

3. Health-related states and events refer to health outcomes of communicable and non-communicable diseases, occupational health, environmental health, mental health, maternal-child health, congenital anomalies, accidents, injuries, *etc*. However, the outcome could be a positive outcome (recovery, survival, reduced risk, access, and utilisation of health services) or a negative outcome (illness, disability, or death).

In applied epidemiology, a study population could be a specific group of patients in a hospital, school pupils, health workers, or factory workers. In epidemiological research, a population could be a particular class of people selected from a specific place and time. Furthermore, this set of people could be categorised based on age, gender, or ethnicity. The structures of populations vary between geographical areas and time. However, such variations must be factored in when conducting analyses to have a clearer picture of what is being studied for inference to be drawn at the end.

It is essential to underscore that the critical tasks in applied epidemiology are public health surveillance, field investigation, analytical studies, evaluation, linkages, and policy development.[3] It suggests that an epidemiologist must be able to effectively create a study design, develop data collection tools, conduct the study, analyse the results, and interpret the findings. Similarly, he must be skilled in data management and interpretation andmust be able to generate reports and disseminate the findings to a broader audience [17, 18].

DIFFERENT FIELDS OF EPIDEMIOLOGY

Epidemiology depends much on understanding disease causation, its transmission, outbreak investigations, and effective disease surveillance. There are clinical epidemiologists, environmental epidemiologists, forensic epidemiologists, occupational epidemiologists, infectious disease epidemiologists, and molecular epidemiologists, to mention but a few, to look at the causes of disease, causality, or associations depending on the setting and the increasing applicability of epidemiology. Here are some of the various fields and subfields of epidemiology:

1. Clinical Epidemiology focuses on issues relevant to clinical medicine. Clinical epidemiologists use clinical trials of drugs to know their efficacy and to monitor the side effects to reduce the number of adverse health outcomes in patients [20, 21].

2. Infectious Disease Epidemiology establishes disease patterns through monitoring and tracking the spread of infectious diseases to observe and predict outbreaks, epidemics, and pandemics. Infectious disease epidemiologists use the outcome of their studies to advise governments and policymakers to put in place measures that mitigate health events. In this area, epidemiologists often work on outbreaks, vaccine development, and strategies to prevent the spread of infections [22].

3. Environmental Epidemiology examines how the environment has harmful consequences on human health. In addition to assessing the impact of human exposure to specific environmental hazards, environmental epidemiologists seek to understand the relationship between external risk factors and disease, illness, injury, developmental abnormalities, or death. They study the relationship between environmental exposures (such as air and water quality, toxins, and pollutants) and health outcomes. They assess the impact of environmental factors on diseases like asthma, cancer, and congenital disabilities [23].

4. Forensic Epidemiology helps fill the gap between clinical judgment and epidemiologic data to establish lawsuit causality. It suffices to say that forensic epidemiologists combine forensic medicine and epidemiology, playing an essential role in civil, criminal, or both lawsuits [24].

5. Occupational Epidemiology investigates workers and their workplace, their health outcomes vis-à-vis causal association with the conditions of the area they operate, such as chemicals, pollutants, radiation, heat, and work schedules, to mention but a few. They study occupational hazards, exposure to harmful substances, and work-related injuries and illnesses [25].

6. Molecular Epidemiology, which emerges from molecular biology, studies the contribution of genetic and environmental risk factors at a molecular level. It enables molecular epidemiologists to understand disease causation, distribution, and prevention within families and across populations. Similarly, it helps in understanding the interactions between genetic traits and environmental exposures in disease causation and the specific molecular and genetic pathways in developing disease. They use genetic and molecular techniques to investigate disease outbreaks and patterns. They often work at the intersection of genetics, epidemiology, and microbiology [26 - 29].

Similarly, there are other fields and subfields within epidemiology, each with a unique focus and methodology. These include chronic disease epidemiology, social epidemiology, reproductive and perinatal epidemiology, nutritional epidemiology, genetic epidemiology, pharmacoepidemiology, cancer epidemiology, global health epidemiology, veterinary epidemiology, and psychiatric epidemiology. Epidemiologists in various areas work to better understand and improve public health by identifying risk factors, developing prevention strategies, and informing healthcare policies and practices.

EPIDEMIOLOGICAL RESEARCH AND METHODS

Epidemiological research employs various paradigms, which include overarching frameworks that guide the design and conduct of studies [30]. These paradigms help epidemiologists structure their investigations and answer specific research questions:

1. Descriptive Epidemiology: This paradigm focuses on characterizing the distribution of diseases or health events in populations. Descriptive studies aim to answer the "who, what, when, and where" questions. They provide essential information about the patterns and trends of diseases.

2. Analytical Epidemiology: Analytical studies go beyond describing disease patterns. They aim to identify the causes of disease and assess the associations between risk factors and health outcomes. Analytical epidemiology addresses the "how" and "why" questions.

3. Experimental Epidemiology: In experimental epidemiology, researchers conduct controlled experiments to investigate the effects of interventions or treatments on health outcomes. Randomized controlled trials (RCTs) are a common example of experimental epidemiological studies.

Types of Epidemiologic Studies

Epidemiologists employ various types of studies to explore health-related questions and draw conclusions about causation.[31]The examples of these studies are:

1. Cross-Sectional Studies: These studies examine the health status and exposure of a population at a single point in time. They are useful for identifying associations but cannot establish causation.

2. Case-Control Studies: Case-control studies compare individuals with a specific disease (case) to those without the disease (control). Researchers assess past exposures to determine potential risk factors.

3. Cohort Studies: Cohort studies follow a group of individuals over time to observe their health outcomes and exposures. They are valuable for assessing causation and determining relative risks.

4. Intervention Studies (Clinical Trials): Intervention studies involve experimental manipulation of a factor to assess its impact on health outcomes. Randomized controlled trials (RCTs) are the gold standard for intervention studies.

5. Ecological Studies: Ecological studies analyze data at the population level, examining associations between group-level exposures and outcomes. They are suitable for generating hypotheses but have limitations in establishing causation at the individual level.

Exercise 3: Designing an Epidemiological Study for Your Community

This exercise will allow readers to gain practical experience in designing an epidemiological study tailored to the unique health concerns of their community, reinforcing their understanding of epidemiological research methods and their applications. Now, let us engage in an exercise to guide readers about designing an epidemiological study for their community:

i. **Select a Research Question**: Identify a health-related research question or issue that is relevant to your community. Consider factors, such as disease prevalence, local concerns, or emerging health challenges.

ii. **Choose a Study Type:** Based on your research questions, decide which type of epidemiological study would be most appropriate. Consider whether a cross-sectional study, case-control study, cohort study, or another design aligns with your objectives.

iii. **Define Study Objectives:** Clearly state the objectives of your study. What specific information are you seeking to uncover? What outcomes or exposures will you investigate?

iv. **Select Your Study Population:** Define the population from which you will draw your study participants. Consider factors like age, gender, location, or other relevant demographics.

v. **Determine Data Collection Methods:** Outline the methods you will use to collect data, including surveys, interviews, medical records, or existing databases. Ensure that your data collection tools are valid and reliable.

vi. **Ethical Considerations:** Address ethical considerations, including informed consent, privacy, and data protection. Ensure that your study complies with ethical guidelines and regulations.

vii. **Data Analysis Plan:** Describe how you plan to analyze the data you collect. Specify the statistical methods or analytical approaches you will use to draw conclusions.

viii. **Budget and Resources:** Consider the resources, funding, and personnel required to conduct your study. Create a preliminary budget and identify potential sources of funding.

ix. *Timeline:Develop a timeline outlining the key milestones and deadlines for your study, from study design to data analysis and reporting.*

x. *Community Engagement:Discuss how you will engage with the community during the study, including communication and dissemination of findings.*

MEASURING DISEASE OCCURRENCE

Disease Frequency and Patterns

Understanding disease occurrence is a central aspect of epidemiology. It involves quantifying the frequency of diseases within a population, identifying patterns, and assessing the burden of health conditions. To achieve this, epidemiologists employ various measures and formulas [32 - 35].

Key Measures and Formulas

1. *Incidence*: Incidence refers to the number of new cases of a disease that develop in a specific population during a defined time period. It provides information about the risk of contracting the disease. There are two types of Incidence: Incidence Rate (IR) and Cumulative Incidence (CI).

Incidence Rate (IR) = (Number of New Cases) / (Population at Risk) x (period)

- Person-time refers to the sum of time-period where each individual in the population was at risk of developing the disease.
- This rate is often expressed per 1,000 or 100,000 person-years.

Example of Incidence Rate: If 150 new cases of a disease are diagnosed in a population of 10,000 people over 2 years, the incidence rate could be calculated as:

IR = 150 / 10,000 x 2 = 150/20,000 = 7.5 per 1,000 persons-years

Cumulative Incidence (CI) = Number of New Cases during a specific period / Total population at risk at the start of the period.

- It is often used for closed populations (where the population at risk remains the same during the study period).
- CI gives a probability estimate of developing the disease over a specified period.

Example of Cumulative Incidence: In a cohort of 5,000 individuals, if 100 people develop the disease over 10 years, the CR could be calculated as:

CI = 100 new cases / 5,000 at risk = 0.02 or 2% over 10 years

2. *Prevalence:* Prevalence refers to the total number of cases (both new and pre-existing) of a disease in a population at a specific point in time or over a period. There are two types of Prevalence: Point Prevalence (PP) and Period Prevalence (PeP).

Point Prevalence = Number of existing cases at a specific point in time / Total population at that time

- The PP provides a snapshot of the disease burden at a specific moment.

Example of Point Prevalence (PP): If a survey on January 1st finds that 300 out of 10,000 people have a certain chronic disease, thenthe PP could be calculated as:

Point Prevalence (PP) = 300 / 10,000 = 0.03 or 3%

Period Prevalence = Number of existing cases during a period / Total population during that period

- The PeP measure accounts for all cases observed over a specified time period.

Example of Period Prevalence (PeP): If in a year, 500 people are observed to have a disease at any point in time within a population of 20,000:

Period Prevalence (PeP) = 500/20,000 = 0.025 or 2.5%

3. *Mortality Rate:* The mortality rate assesses the number of deaths from a specific disease within a population over a defined period. It is calculated using the formula:

Mortality Rate = (Number of Deaths from Disease) / (Total Population) x 1000 (or 100,000, depending on the population size).

Example of Mortality Rate: *In a town with a population of 50,000 people, if there were 200 deaths due to a specific disease in a given year, then the mortality rate could be calculated as:*

Mortality Rate (MR) = (Number of Deaths from Disease) / (Total Population) × 1000

Mortality Rate (MR): (200/50,000) × 1000 = 200/50 = 4 deaths per 1,000 people

4. Attack Rate: *The attack rate is useful in outbreak investigations and measures the proportion of a population that becomes ill after exposure to a specific agent. It is calculated using the formula:*

Attack Rate = (Number of Cases) / (Number of People Exposed) x 100

Example of Attack Rate:*In a school with 1,000 students, there was an outbreak of influenza. Out of the 1,000 students, 150 got infected with the flu. Then, the attack rate could be calculated as:*

Attack Rate (AR) = (150/1000) × 100 = 15%

In this example, the attack rate is 15%, meaning 15% of the exposed population (students) became infected during the outbreak.

Exercise 4: Calculating Disease Rates for Local Health Issues

This exercise encourages readers to actively apply epidemiological measures to a real-world scenario, fostering a deeper understanding of disease occurrence and its relevance to local health challenges. In this exercise, readers will apply their knowledge of disease occurrence measures to calculate disease rates for local health issues:

   i. **Select a Local Health Issue:** Choose a specific health issue or disease that is relevant to your community. Consider factors, such as prevalence, incidence, or mortality rates related to this issue.
   ii. **Gather Data:** Collect relevant data, including the number of cases or deaths attributed to the health issue within your community, as well as the total population at risk and the period of interest.
   iii. **Calculate Incidence Rate:** If applicable, calculate the incidence rate for the chosen health issue using the provided formula. This will help you understand how quickly new cases are emerging.
   iv. ***Calculate Prevalence:****Calculate the prevalence of the health issue within your community using the formula. This will provide insight into the overall burden of the condition.*
   v. ***Determine Mortality Rate:****If relevant, calculate the mortality rate associated with the health issue. This will help you assess the impact on the population.*
   vi. ***Assess Trends:****Analyze the calculated rates and trends over time. Consider any variations or patterns that emerge from the data.*
   vii. ***Interpret Findings:****Interpret your findings. What do the calculated rates tell you about the impact of health issues on your community? Are there disparities among different demographic groups?*
   viii. *Discuss Implications: Discuss the implications of your findings for local health policy and interventions. How can the data inform public health strategies to address the health issue?*

USES, TRIUMPHS, AND APPLICATIONS

Epidemiology aims to enhance the health of the populace by generating information that helps clinicians, policy, and decision-makers. Through a systematic approach, epidemiologists assess and answer these questions on the state of health of a population: What, Who, Where, When, and Why/How. Epidemiology is the cornerstone of public health because it plays a critical role in understanding the distribution and determinants of health-related events in populations. Its applications are vast and multifaceted, and it contributes significantly to the advancement of public health. It is important to underscore that one of the primary applications of epidemiology is in disease surveillance [1 - 4, 7, 12, 16, 36]. By monitoring the occurrence of diseases within populations, epidemiologists can identify trends, detect outbreaks, and initiate timely interventions. This proactive approach is fundamental in controlling the spread of infectious diseases and mitigating their impact on communities.

Similarly, epidemiology informs policy development and health planning. By analyzing data on the prevalence, incidence, and risk factors of diseases, public health officials can develop targeted interventions and allocate resources more effectively. This evidence-based decision-making ensures that health programs are both efficient and impactful.

Epidemiology also plays a critical role in the evaluation of public health interventions. By assessing the effectiveness of vaccination programs, health campaigns, and other interventions, epidemiologists help ensure that these efforts achieve their intended outcomes. This continuous feedback loop allows for the refinement of strategies, leading to improved health outcomes over time [1 - 4, 7, 12, 16, 36].

In the realm of research, epidemiology provides the foundation for identifying risk factors for disease and potential targets for intervention. Through cohort studies, case-control studies, and randomized controlled trials, epidemiologists contribute to the understanding of the causes of diseases and the development of new treatments and prevention strategies. The benefits of epidemiology for public health are profound. By identifying the factors that contribute to disease and injury, epidemiology helps prevent illness and promote health. It provides the data necessary to implement public health policies, design effective health programs, and respond to emerging health threats. In essence, epidemiology is indispensable for the protection and improvement of population health, making it a fundamental tool in the pursuit of global health equity and well-being. Epidemiology, considered as a tool for the improvement of the health of the public, could be used to help in the following areas [1 - 3, 12, 16, 36]:

- Assess the health of a community to help policy and decision-makers develop guidelines frameworks, set goals, and monitor progress in their implementation.
- Search for the causes of a disease.
- Describe the health status of the population or groups.
- Discover and bridge gaps in the natural history of diseases.
- Disease control to break the weakest link in the chain of transmission of communicable diseases and reduce non-communicable diseases.
- Evaluate health programs and interventions.
- Determine the chances or probability of occurrence of disease/death and disability.
- Adequately manage health and hospital services.
- Set cut-off levels between normal and abnormal populations and establish trigger levels for action or intervention.

The historical achievements of epidemiology started in the late 19th century when disease association with causal factors and disease eradication was proven to be possible. Although there are several triumphs of epidemiology, some of them discussed below include smallpox eradication, the causal link between cigarette smoking/asbestos and lung cancer, rheumatic fever/heart disease and poverty, methyl mercury poisoning from consumption of contaminated fish, iodine deficiency and goitre, to mention a few. However, there is a need to underscore that the challenges in modern epidemiology are enormous. As mentioned earlier, in addition to emerging or reemerging infectious disease agents, biological warfare and bioterrorism are increasingly posing additional threats to global peace [2, 16, 18]. The globalized world has been faced with a succession of diseases that rapidly spread across the globe, which include the AIDS pandemic, the SARS outbreak, the influenza pandemic, the Ebola outbreak, the Zika virus, and the COVID-19 pandemic. These have shown that all countries are vulnerable and further exposed the weaknesses of the global disease surveillance platform and health systems, as well as the reluctance of countries to monitor and report accordingly.

These factors, along with others,have resulted in the world desperate for reform in global health leadership, echoing a call for effective global health governance [37, 38]. Nonetheless, some of the historical achievements of epidemiology include the following:

Smallpox eradication: The milestone achievements of the historic eradication of smallpox through applied epidemiology only came to the fore in 1980; this is 180 years after the development of the smallpox vaccine by Edward Jenner for cowpox infection. The 10-year eradication plan, spearheaded by the WHO in its 10-year plan (1967 – 76), decreased cases and deaths from 31 countries to only 2 in 1976. This giant stride became possible by understanding the epidemiology of the disease, innovative approaches of epidemiologists to herd immunity, and, most importantly, the collaboration of countries worldwide. In addition to universal political will and government commitment, epidemiologists established the absence of non-human reservoirs of the disease or subclinical carriers and the conferment of life-long immunity in survivors [12, 39].

Methyl mercury poisoning: In the 1950s, mercury compounds discharged into a river from a factory in Minamata, Japan, resulted in environmental pollution and caused severe methyl mercury poisoning in people who consumed fish. It was estimated that at least 50,000 people were affected with at least 2,000 cases of Minamata disease. The Minamata disease, which resulted from consuming fish polluted by methylmercury, was discovered through applied observational epidemiological studies. Some countries also reported a lighter form of the disease, all attributed to consuming fish contaminated by methylmercury [40 - 42].

Rheumatic fever and rheumatic heart disease: Epidemiological studies highlighted the association between rheumatic fever (and rheumatic heart disease), caused by infection with a streptococcal organism, and multiple factors, such as poverty, overcrowding, poor housing, and poor socioeconomic condition. However, based on the recommendations of epidemiologists to improve the socioeconomic status and living conditions of the populace, the disease started to disappear [43, 44].

Goitre and iodine deficiency: Although first described 400 years ago, this disease was only discovered to be associated with iodine deficiency in the twentieth century. In 1915, goitre was realized to be a preventable disease through epidemiological studies. History has it that Switzerland was the first country to propose using iodized salt to address the scourge, which was subsequently scaled up for large-scale community use across the globe [41, 45].

Lung cancer and cigarette smoking/Asbestos dust: It was after 1930 that the dramatic increase of a disease that was hitherto rare led epidemiologists to study the causal association between lung cancer and tobacco users. It was in 1950 that studies linking lung cancer with tobacco use were first published. Similarly, additional epidemiological studies showed that exposure to other carcinogenic substances, such as asbestos and urban air pollutants, was associated with increased lung cancer burden; the studies also proved the multiplicative effect of carcinogenic substances when combined with cigarette smoking [46, 47].

CONCLUSION

In conclusion, Chapter 1 serves as an indispensable primer on the foundations of epidemiology. By unravelling the complexities of health and disease, delineating different fields, and elucidating research methodologies, the chapter equips readers with a solid footing in epidemiological concepts. Furthermore, it underscores the practical applications and triumphs of epidemiology, reinforcing its pivotal role in shaping public health policies, disease prevention strategies, and healthcare interventions. As readers progress through subsequent chapters, they will continue to build upon these foundational principles, gaining deeper insights into the dynamic and indispensable field of epidemiology.

REFERENCES

[1]   Wallace RB. Maxcy-Rosenau-Last Public Health and Preventive Medicine. 14th ed., Norwalk, Connecticut: Appleton & Lange 1998.

[2]   Oakley A. Fifty years of JN Morris's Uses of Epidemiology. Int J Epidemiol 2007; 36(6): 1184-5. [http://dx.doi.org/10.1093/ije/dym230] [PMID: 18056127]

[3]   Last JM. A dictionary of epidemiology. Oxford University Press 2001.

[4]   Rothman KJ, Greenland S, Lash TL. Modern epidemiology. Lippincott Williams & Wilkins 2008.

[5]   Checkoway H, Pearce N, Kriebel D. Research Methods in Occupational Epidemiology. 2nd ed., Oxford University Press 2004. [http://dx.doi.org/10.1093/acprof:oso/9780195092424.001.0001]

[6]   Johnson S. The Ghost Map: The Story of London's Most Terrifying Epidemic—and How It Changed Science, Cities, and the Modern World. Riverhead Books 2006.

[7]   Lee LM, Thacker SB, St. Louis ME. Principles & Practice of Public Health Surveillance. 3rd ed., Oxford University Press 2010. [http://dx.doi.org/10.1093/acprof:oso/9780195372922.001.0001]

[8]   Tulchinsky T H. John Snow, Cholera, the Broad Street Pump; Waterborne Diseases Then and Now. Case Studies in Public Health 2018; 77-99. [http://dx.doi.org/10.1016/B978-0-12-804571-8.00017-2]

[9]   WHO. Cholera Annual Report 2017. Weekly Epidemiological Record 21 September 2018; 93(38): pp 489-500. Available from: http://www.who.int/wer/2018/wer9338/en/

[10]   Thun MJ, Carter BD, Feskanich D, *et al.* 50-year trends in smoking-related mortality in the United States. N Engl J Med 2013; 368(4): 351-64. [http://dx.doi.org/10.1056/NEJMsa1211127] [PMID: 23343064]

[11]   Kannel WB. The Framingham Study: ITS 50-year legacy and future promise. J Atheroscler Thromb 2000; 6(2): 60-6. [http://dx.doi.org/10.5551/jat1994.6.60] [PMID: 10872616]

[12]   Bhattacharya S. Expunging Variola: The Control and Eradication of Smallpox in India, 1947–1977. Orient BlackSwan 2019.

[13]   Zimmern RL. Genetics in disease prevention.Oxford Handbook of Public Health Practice. Oxford: Oxford University Press 2001; pp. 544-9.

[14]   Moore ZS, Seward JF, Lane JM. Smallpox. Lancet 2006; 367(9508): 425-35. [http://dx.doi.org/10.1016/S0140-6736(06)68143-9] [PMID: 16458769]

[15]   Pennington H. Smallpox and bioterrorism. Bull World Health Organ 2003; 81(10): 762-7.
       [PMID: 14758439]

[16]   Bonita R, Beaglehole R, Kjellström T. Basic epidemiology. 2nd ed., World Health Organ 2006.

[17]   An Introduction to Applied Epidemiology and Biostatistics.Principles of Epidemiology in Public
       Health Practice. 3rd ed. Atlanta, GA: Centers for Disease Control and Prevention 2012; p. 30333.

[18]   WHO. COVID-19 Pandemic. 2020. Avaiable from: https://www.who.int/emergencies/diseases/novel-
       coronavirus-2019/events-as-they-happen

[19]   Huber M, Knottnerus JA, Green L, *et al.* How should we define health? BMJ 2011; 343(jul26 2):
       d4163.
       [http://dx.doi.org/10.1136/bmj.d4163] [PMID: 21791490]

[20]   Fletcher RH, Fletcher SW, Fletcher GS. Clinical Epidemiology: The Essentials. 5th ed., Lippincott
       Williams & Wilkins 2014.

[21]   Rothman KJ, Greenland S, Lash T. Modern epidemiology. 3rd ed. Philadelphia: Lippincott Williams
       & Wilkins 2008; pp. 303-27.

[22]   Barreto ML, Teixeira MG, Carmo EH. Infectious diseases epidemiology. J Epidemiol Community
       Health 2006; 60(3): 192-5.
       [http://dx.doi.org/10.1136/jech.2003.011593] [PMID: 16476746]

[23]   Merrill RM. Environmental epidemiology: principles and methods. Sudbury, Mass.: Jones and Bartlett
       Publishers 2008; pp. 8-9.

[24]   Michael F, Maurice Z. Forensic Epidemiology: Principles and Practices. Elsevier 2016.

[25]   Harvey C, Neil P, David L. Research Methods in Occupational Epidemiology. New York, NY: Oxford
       University Press 2004.

[26]   Porta M, Greenland S, Hernán M, dos Santos Silva I, Last JM. A dictionary of epidemiology. 6th ed.,
       New York: Oxford University Press 2014.
       [http://dx.doi.org/10.1093/acref/9780199976720.001.0001]

[27]   Kilbourne ED. The molecular epidemiology of influenza. J Infect Dis 1973; 127(4): 478-87.
       [http://dx.doi.org/10.1093/infdis/127.4.478] [PMID: 4121053]

[28]   Porta M, Malats N, Vioque J, *et al.* Incomplete overlapping of biological, clinical, and environmental
       information in molecular epidemiological studies: a variety of causes and a cascade of consequences. J
       Epidemiol Community Health 2002; 56(10): 734-8.
       [http://dx.doi.org/10.1136/jech.56.10.734] [PMID: 12239196]

[29]   Wild CP, Vineis P, Garte S. Molecular Epidemiology of Chronic Diseases. 1st ed., Wiley-Blackwell
       2011.

[30]   Porta M. A dictionary of epidemiology. 6th ed., Oxford University Press 2014.
       [http://dx.doi.org/10.1093/acref/9780199976720.001.0001]

[31]   Ahlbom A. Williams & Wilkins. 2021.Modern Epidemiology.
       [http://dx.doi.org/10.1007/s10654-021-00778-w]

[32]   Kleinbaum DG, Klein M. Survival analysis: A self-learning text. Springer Science & Business Media
       2010.

[33]   Bosman A. Incubation period, Latent period and Generation time. European Centre for Disease
       Prevention and Control 2012.

[34]   Hernandez JBR, Kim PY. Epidemiology Morbidity And Mortality. Treasure Island, FL: StatPearls
       Publishing LLC 2020.

[35]   Alexander LK, Lope B, Ricchetti-Masterson K, Yeatts KB. Calculating Person-Time Eric Notebook.
       2nd ed., The University of North Carolina 2015.https://sph.unc.edu/files/2015/07/nciph_ERIC4.pdf

[36]   Kamps BS, Hoffmann C. SARS Reference. 3rd ed., Flying Publisher 2003.
       http://www.sarsreference.com/index.htm

[37]   Koplan JP, Bond TC, Merson MH, *et al.* Towards a common definition of global health. Lancet 2009;
       373(9679): 1993-5.
       [http://dx.doi.org/10.1016/S0140-6736(09)60332-9] [PMID: 19493564]

[38]   Smith R, Lee K. Global health governance: we need innovation not renovation. BMJ Glob Health
       2017; 2(2): e000275.
       [http://dx.doi.org/10.1136/bmjgh-2016-000275] [PMID: 28589032]

[39]   WHO. The Smallpox Eradication Programme. 2010; (1966-1980). Avaialble from:
       https://www.who.int/features/2010/smallpox/en/

[40]   McCurry J. Japan remembers Minamata. Lancet 2006; 367(9505): 99-100.
       [http://dx.doi.org/10.1016/S0140-6736(06)67944-0] [PMID: 16419257]

[41]   Methylmercury (Environmental health criteria, No101). Geneva: World Health Organization 1990.

[42]   Children's Exposure to Mercury Compounds. Geneva, Switzerland: WHO Document Production
       Services 2010.

[43]   Hajar R. Rheumatic fever and rheumatic heart disease a historical perspective. Heart Views 2016;
       17(3): 120-6.
       [http://dx.doi.org/10.4103/1995-705X.192572] [PMID: 27867464]

[44]   Olivier C. Rheumatic Fever – Is it still a problem? J Antimicrobial Chemotherapy, 45. Topic 2000; T1:
       13-21.

[45]   Zimmermann MB. Research on iodine deficiency and goiter in the 19th and early 20th centuries. J Nutr
       2008; 138(11): 2060-3.
       [http://dx.doi.org/10.1093/jn/138.11.2060] [PMID: 18936198]

[46]   Khang YH. The causality between smoking and lung cancer among groups and individuals: addressing
       issues in tobacco litigation in South Korea. Epidemiol Health 2015; 37: e2015026.
       [http://dx.doi.org/10.4178/epih/e2015026] [PMID: 26137845]

[47]   Thun MJ. When truth is unwelcome: the first reports on smoking and lung cancer. Bull World Health
       Organ 2005; 83(2): 144-5.
       [PMID: 15744407]

CHAPTER 2

Epidemiological Models and Frameworks

Abstract: Chapter 2 delves into the conceptual frameworks and models that underpin epidemiological analysis and understanding. Beginning with an introduction to the themes of the chapter, it explores foundational models, such as the Epidemiologic Triad and the chain of infection. The chapter elucidates the natural history of the disease and presents various epidemiological frameworks used to study and interpret disease dynamics. Through a comprehensive examination of these models and frameworks, readers gain a deeper appreciation of the conceptual tools essential for epidemiological inquiry.

Keywords: Epidemiological Models, Epidemiologic Triad, Chain of Infection, Natural History of Disease, Frameworks, Disease Dynamics.

INTRODUCTION

In the vast tapestry of human existence, few forces have shaped our destiny as profoundly as infectious diseases. From the plagues of antiquity to the ongoing battle against global pandemics, these invisible adversaries have challenged our resilience, adaptability, and scientific prowess. In Chapter 1, we delve into the history of epidemiology, tracing its evolution from ancient civilizations to the modern era. Now, as we venture deeper into the heart of the subject, we confront the very tools that have empowered us to understand, predict, and combat infectious diseases - Epidemiological Models and frameworks [1].

Epidemiological models are the intellectual scaffolding upon which the edifice of epidemiology stands. They are the compass that guides us through the complex terrain of disease transmission, helping us decipher the cryptic patterns of contagion and evaluate the impact of interventions. In this chapter, we embark on a journey into the world of epidemiological modelling, seeking to demystify these intricate constructs and unveil their role in shaping our understanding of disease dynamics [1, 2].

Our exploration begins with an examination of the fundamental principles that underpin epidemiological models. We will unravel the mathematical equations and conceptual frameworks that give life to these models, making them powerful instruments for simulating the spread of diseases. As we delve into their inner workings, the reader will gain a profound appreciation for the elegance and precision with which these models capture the essence of epidemics [1, 2].

However, models are not static entities; they are dynamic tools that evolve alongside our knowledge and technological capabilities. Hence, this chapter will also explore cutting-edge developments and innovations in epidemiological modelling. From agent-based simulations that mimic individual behaviours to advanced machine learning techniques that enhance our predictive capabilities, we will witness how epidemiology constantly evolves in the face of new challenges [1 - 3].

As we navigate the intricacies of epidemiological models and frameworks, it is essential to remember that these tools are not mere abstractions. They hold the power to inform public health policy, guide resource allocation, and ultimately save lives. In understanding them, we equip ourselves with the means to make informed decisions in an increasingly interconnected world where the threat of infectious diseases knows no borders [1 - 4].

So, let us embark on this intellectual voyage into the heart of epidemiology, where we will unravel the mathematical tapestry of disease transmission, explore the innovative frontiers of modelling, and discover how these tools empower us to confront the ever-evolving challenges of infectious diseases. Welcome to Chapter 2 of our journey, where we dive deep into the world of Epidemiological Models and frameworks.

THE EPIDEMIOLOGIC TRIAD

Agent, Host, and Environment

As we all know, epidemiology is one crucial tool that studies the influence of the environment on human health. It is critical to underscore that some diseases have genetic influence, especially when interacting with environmental factors (biological, chemical, physical, psychosocial, economic, and cultural). Similarly, epidemiologists understand that no single disease causation model adequately explains the concept of disease causation and other health events in a population. However, various diseases occur because of an interplay between several factors. There are two most common models that try to explain disease causation: the epidemiologic triad, also called a traditional model for infectious diseases (agent, susceptible host, and environment), and the causal pie model for non-infectious diseases, which was proposed by Rothman in 1976 [1, 2].

The Epidemiologic Triad model is a foundational concept in epidemiology that helps us understand the complex interplay of factors contributing to disease occurrence. The model consists of three key components - an agent, a susceptible host, and the environment.

1. *Agent*: The agent refers to the microorganism, substance, or factor responsible for causing the disease. Agents can be infectious microorganisms like bacteria, viruses, or parasites, or they can be non-infectious factors, such as chemicals, toxins, or genetic mutations. If the disease agent is infectious, consideration should be given to the virulence, pathogenicity, and infectivity/infective dose. However, while the epidemiologic triad works out well for some diseases, it has its limitations for cardiovascular diseases, cancer, or other diseases that have other associated causative factors [3 - 5].

- **Dominance of the Agent:** In some diseases, the agent plays a dominant role in determining the course of the disease. For instance, the virulence of the *Mycobacterium tuberculosis* bacterium is crucial in tuberculosis, where the ability of the pathogen to evade the immune system can lead to chronic infection.
- **Examples:**
- **Influenza Virus:** The agent is a virus with high infectivity, capable of causing seasonal epidemics and pandemics.
- **Plasmodium Parasite:** In malaria, the *Plasmodium* species acts as the agent, with its lifecycle intricately tied to the host and the environment.

2. *Host*: The host represents the individual or population susceptible to the disease. Host susceptibility varies among individuals and populations, and host factors include intrinsic (*e.g.*, genetic predisposition, age, sex, immune status, and other biological characteristics) or extrinsic (*e.g.*, social lifestyle, occupation, hygiene, culture) factors of the host, as they influence the outcome of the host-agent interactions [3 - 5].

- **Dominance of the Host:** In some diseases, host factors play a significant role. For example, genetic predispositions can make certain individuals more susceptible to diseases like sickle cell anaemia or cystic fibrosis, where the genetic profile of the host is a primary determinant of disease manifestation.
- **Examples:**
- **HIV Infection:** The immune status of the host is crucial, with the virus exploiting its immune cells, leading to immunodeficiency.
- **Sickle Cell Disease:** A genetic mutation in the host causes the disease, independent of any external agent or environmental factors.

3. *Environment*: The environment encompasses the external factors and conditions influencing disease transmission and progression. Environmental factors can include physical conditions (temperature, humidity), social and cultural factors (socioeconomic status, living conditions), ecological factors (animal reservoirs, vectors), and availability and accessibility of health services [3 - 5].

- **Dominance of the Environment:** Environmental factors can sometimes be the most critical element in disease causation. For instance, in vector-borne diseases like malaria, the presence of suitable mosquito breeding sites (standing water) is a dominant environmental factor.
- **Examples:**
- **Malaria:** The environment plays a critical role, as the presence of Anopheles mosquitoes, climatic conditions, and human activities such as agriculture can significantly affect disease transmission.
- **Cholera:** Contaminated water sources in the environment are crucial in the spread of *Vibrio cholerae*, the agent causing cholera.

However, the risk factors in the Epidemiologic Triad are not distributed randomly in a population, resulting in some individuals being more likely to manifest a disease than others; hence, there is a need to identify those factors that place some people at greater risk than others. This traditional model fits in well for infectious diseases and is also referred to as the epidemiologic triangle (Fig. **1**) [1, 2].

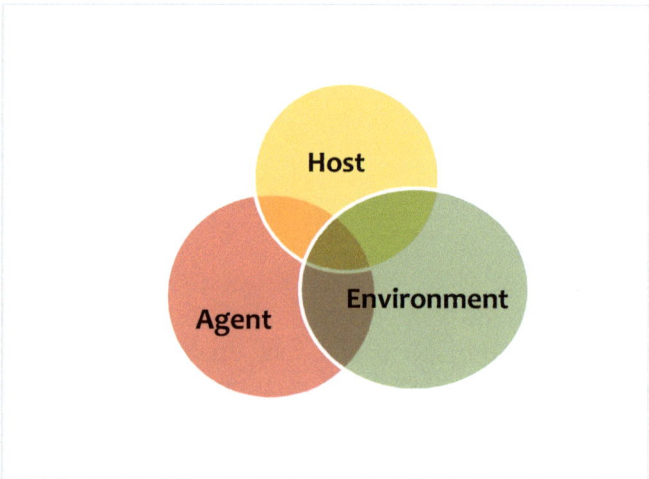

Fig. (1). Epidemiologic triad model.

Interaction Between Agent, Host, and Environment

The interaction between the agent, host, and environment determines whether a disease occurs and how it progresses. A change in any one of these components can disrupt the balance and lead to the emergence or re-emergence of diseases. For example, deforestation (environment) can bring humans (host) into closer contact with wildlife, leading to the spillover of zoonotic diseases (agents) [3 - 5].

Classical Epidemiological Theory vs. Other Theories of Disease Causation

Classical epidemiological theory, as illustrated by the Epidemiologic Triad, focuses on the interaction between the agent, host, and environment. This model is effective for infectious diseases, where the relationship between these three elements is clear and direct [3 - 5]. However, with the emergence of chronic diseases and a deeper understanding of complex disease mechanisms, other theories have been developed to explain disease causation:

Web of Causation

This theory posits that disease is rarely the result of a single factor. Instead, it is the outcome of a complex interaction of multiple factors, including genetic, environmental, social, and behavioural factors. The Web of Causation is particularly useful for understanding chronic diseases like cardiovascular disease, cancer, and diabetes, where multiple risk factors contribute to disease onset and progression [3 - 5].

Social Determinants of Health

This framework emphasizes the role of social, economic, and political factors in disease causation. It argues that health disparities are largely driven by unequal access to resources, education, and healthcare, as well as by social and cultural practices. This approach is critical for addressing public health issues that are rooted in social inequalities [3 - 5].

Eco-Epidemiology

Eco-epidemiology integrates ecological principles into epidemiology, focusing on the interactions between human populations, their environments, and disease. It is particularly relevant for understanding diseases influenced by environmental changes, such as those related to climate change or urbanization [3 - 5].

Genetic Epidemiology

This branch of epidemiology focuses on the role of genetic factors in health and disease. It involves studying the distribution of genes and their association with diseases within populations. Genetic epidemiology is essential for understanding hereditary diseases and the genetic predisposition to common diseases like hypertension and diabetes.

In summary, while the classical Epidemiologic Triad provides a foundational framework for understanding disease causation, modern epidemiology recognizes the complexity of disease processes and incorporates multiple theories to explain the multifaceted interactions that contribute to health and disease [3 - 5].

Applying the Triad to Disease Causation

Understanding disease causation requires considering how these three components interact. Diseases often result from the dynamic interplay of agents, hosts, and environmental factors [3, 4]. Here is how the triad applies to disease causation:

1. *Direct Causation:* A specific agent sometimes causes a disease in a susceptible host under particular environmental conditions. For example, the influenza virus (agent) can cause flu symptoms in individuals with compromised immune systems (host) during the flu season (environment).

2. *Indirect Causation*: In other instances, disease causation is more complex and may involve multiple factors. Genetic predisposition, lifestyle choices, and exposure to environmental factors can influence the susceptibility of a host. For instance, lung cancer (disease) can result from the interaction of smoking (environment), genetic susceptibility (host), and exposure to carcinogens (agents).

3. *Multifactorial Causation:* Many diseases have multifactorial causation, involving a combination of agents, host factors, and environmental influences. Chronic diseases like heart disease, diabetes, and cancer often fall into this category.

This interaction, referred to as the *Causal Pie model,* was first proposed by Rothman in 1976. It considers the multifactorial nature of disease causation, especially for non-infectious diseases. It is a pie illustration, and a disease occurs when the individual factors come together. These factors are referred to individually as component causes (A, B, C, D, E), and upon coming together, they form a sufficient cause (Fig. **2**) [3]. It is critical to note that a component cause can be any epidemiologic triad model (agent, host, or environment). When a particular component cause is required in a pie before the disease sets in, a particular component cause is a necessary cause. For example, if someone is to get tuberculosis, that person must be infected with Mycobacterium tuberculosis; the infective agent, in this case, is a necessary cause.

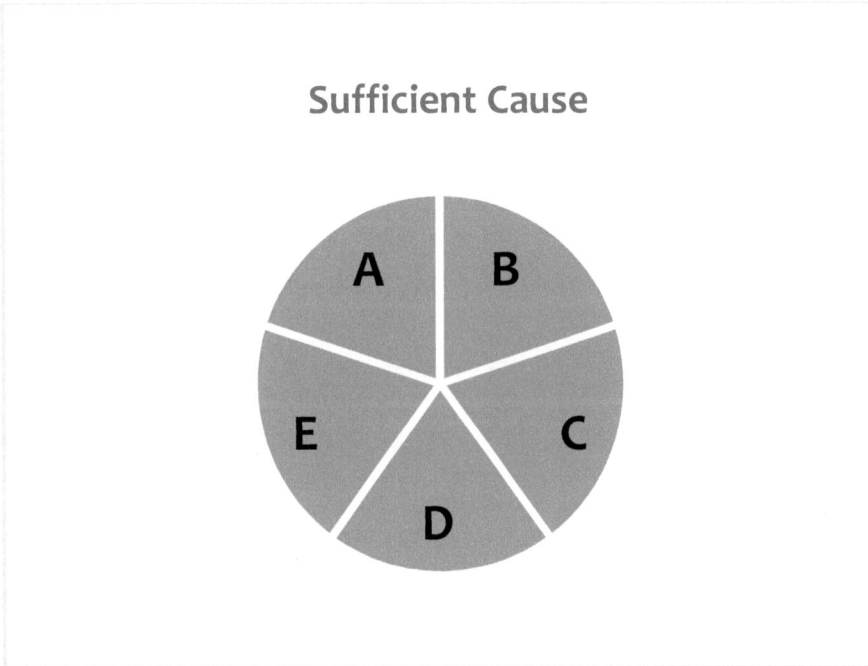

Fig. (2). Causal pie model.

Moreover, a single component cause may not be sufficient to cause a disease. For example, exposure to meningococcal bacteria may not necessarily result in meningitis infection unless the host immunity is compromised. Similarly, a disease could result from more than one sufficient cause (*e.g.*, smoking and asbestos in lung cancer) [3, 4].

Exercise 1: Identifying Local Disease Determinants

In this exercise, readers will apply the concept of the Epidemiologic Triad to identify local disease determinants in their community:

i. **Select a Local Disease**: Choose a specific disease that is relevant to your community. Consider factors, such as disease prevalence, incidence, or public health concerns.

   ii. **Identify Agents, Hosts, and Environmental Factors:** Analyze the causation of disease by breaking it down into its components. Identify the agents responsible for the disease, the characteristics of susceptible hosts, and the environmental factors contributing to its spread.

  iii. **Evaluate Interactions:** Examine how agents, host, and environmental factors interact to influence disease occurrence. Consider how changes in one component may impact disease transmission or severity.

  iv. **Local Context:** Take into account the unique characteristics of your community or region. How do local cultural, socioeconomic, and environmental factors play a role in disease causation?

   v. **Propose Interventions:** Based on your analysis, we propose interventions and strategies to address the identified disease determinants. Consider preventive measures, health education campaigns, or policy changes tailored to the needs of your community.

NB: This exercise encourages readers to apply the Epidemiologic Triad to their local context, helping them identify the complex web of factors influencing disease causation in their community and guiding the development of targeted public health interventions.

THE CHAIN OF INFECTION

Transmission Dynamics

Understanding the chain of infection is crucial for epidemiologists and public health professionals as it provides insights into how infectious diseases are transmitted from one individual to another. The term *chain of infection* is when an infectious microbe leaves its host (reservoir of infection) through a portal of exit and enters into another susceptible host through an ideal portal of entry to cause infection.[3,5,6] The reservoir could be a human, animal (zoonosis), or environment (plants, soil, or water), depending on the case. It is important to note that there are different ways an infectious agent can be transmitted to a susceptible host: direct (direct contact or droplet spread) or indirect (airborne, vehicle-borne, or vector-borne). However, the ability of a host to develop or resist infection depends on intrinsic (*e.g.*, genetic, specific immunity) and extrinsic factors (*e.g.*, malnutrition, alcoholism) [3, 5, 6].

The chain of infection consists of a series of interconnected links, each representing a step in the transmission process. These links include the following:

1. Infectious Agent: This is the microorganism or pathogen responsible for causing the disease. It can be bacteria, viruses, fungi, or parasites.

2. Reservoir: The reservoir is the source of the infectious agent. It can be a human, animal, or environmental source where the pathogen resides and multiplies.

3. Portal of Exit: The pathogen needs a way to exit the body of the reservoir host to infect a new host. Common portals of exit include respiratory secretions (*e.g.*, coughing, sneezing), feces, urine, or blood.

4. Mode of Transmission: This refers to the method by which the pathogen is transferred from the reservoir to a susceptible host. Modes of transmission include direct contact (*e.g.*, person-to-person), indirect contact (*e.g.*, contaminated surfaces), droplet transmission, airborne transmission, vector-borne transmission (*e.g.*, through insects), and more.

5. Portal of Entry: Just as the pathogen needs an exit, it also requires a point of entry into the body of the new host. Entry points can be through the respiratory tract, gastrointestinal tract, mucous membranes, or breaks in the skin.

6. Susceptible Host: The final link in the chain is the individual who is vulnerable to infection. Factors that influence susceptibility include host defence (*e.g.*, immune system), age, overall health, and vaccination status.

Implications for Disease Control

Understanding the chain of infection is instrumental in controlling the spread of infectious diseases. Public health measures target one or more of these links to disrupt the transmission cycle [7]. The examples are as follows:

1. Hand Hygiene: Promoting proper handwashing (removing pathogens from the hands) helps break the chain at the portal of exit and the mode of transmission.

2. Vaccination: Vaccination strengthens host defences, reducing susceptibility and interrupting the chain at the susceptible host link.

3. Quarantine: Isolating infected individuals or animals (reservoir) prevents further transmission to susceptible hosts.

4. Vector Control: Eliminating disease-carrying vectors (*e.g.*, mosquitoes) interrupts the transmission of vector-borne diseases.

The implications of understanding the chain of infection are that it helps determine appropriate control measures using the most cost-effective means. Depending on the disease, an appropriate intervention could be controlling or eliminating the agent at its source – *e.g.*, treatment of a clinical case to eliminate the infection and reduce the risk of transmission, decontamination of soil or vehicle to prevent the escape of an infectious agent, isolation of an infected person to prevent transmission, environment sanitation to prevent faeco-oral transmission, promoting handwashing or use of sanitisers to prevent transmission, adequate air ventilation, and use of masks, prophylactic drugs, and vaccinations [3, 7]. There is also the principle of *herd immunity,* another strategy to prevent a pathogen from encountering a susceptible host to cause an outbreak in a given population. For herd immunity to be of use, at least 80 percent of the population must have some high level of immunity to protect the few susceptible ones. However, the degree of herd immunity required to prevent an outbreak depends on the type of disease (*e.g.*, it works for polio but not for measles and rubella infections). In some diseases, the susceptible ones are often clustered into subgroups based on their cultural or socioeconomic status, and an outbreak ensues [3, 7, 8].

Exercise 2: Tracing the Chain of Infection for Outbreaks

In this exercise, readers will apply their knowledge of the chain of infection to trace the transmission dynamics of a specific outbreak:

   i. **Select an Outbreak**: Choose a recent or historical disease outbreak to investigate. It can be a local or global outbreak.
  ii. **Identify the Chain Links:** Analyze the outbreak by identifying each link in the chain of infection. Determine the infectious agent, reservoir, portal of exit, mode of transmission, portal of entry, and susceptible host.
 iii. **Trace Transmission**: Investigate how the pathogen traveled from the reservoir to the susceptible hosts. Consider factors, such as the mode of transmission and the locations where transmission occurred.
  iv. **Control Measures:** Evaluate the control measures that were implemented to interrupt the chain of infection during the outbreak. Were quarantine measures employed? Was vaccination widely administered?
   v. **Lessons Learned:** Reflect on the effectiveness of the control measures and their impact on containing the outbreak. Consider what lessons can be applied to future disease control efforts.

NB: This exercise allows readers to apply the concept of the chain of infection to real-world outbreaks, enhancing their understanding of how infectious diseases spread and how targeted interventions can be employed for effective disease control.

THE NATURAL HISTORY OF DISEASE

Natural History of the Disease, the Chain of Infection, and its Implications

Epidemiologists are particularly interested in studying the natural history of diseases (course and outcome) in individuals or groups. They leverage this to design studies that enable them to understand disease causation, evaluate interventions (treatments, preventive measures, health promotion), and assess the efficiency of public health services [9].

It all starts with exposure to an infective agent (microorganism) or hazardous substance (*e.g.*, tobacco smoke) over time sufficient to cause disease in a vulnerable host. Once the disease starts, the system undergoes some pathological changes at a subclinical stage. In infectious diseases, the infected individual starts incubating (exposure time to disease onset varies depending on the infective agent). Similarly, this period could last for decades in chronic diseases and is called the latency period.

It is worth mentioning that the incubation period of some acute conditions could range between seconds to minutes (*e.g.*, hypersensitivity or toxic reactions) [14]. Table **1** shows the incubation period, called the latency period. It is also known as the subclinical stage, when pathological changes occur in an individual and can only be picked up using specialized investigations and screening. So, intervening at this stage would save the situation [3, 15].

Table 1. The incubation period of some diseases in humans [10 - 13].

Diseases	Incubation Period
Cholera	12hrs - 5 days
COVID-19	2 - 14 days
Dengue Fever	3 - 14 days
Ebola	1 - 42 days
Influenza	1 - 3 days
Malaria	7 - 30 days
Measles	9 - 12 days
Polio	7 - 14 days
Salmonella	12 - 24 hrs
Tetanus	7 - 21 days
Tuberculosis	2 - 12 weeks
Typhoid	7 - 21 days

The clinical stage sets in once symptoms begin to manifest. These symptoms could range from mild to severe or fatal, as the case may be; this range is referred to as the *spectrum of disease*. The result of the disease process could be recovery, disability, or death (Fig. **3**). However, it is essential to note that some individuals could remain asymptomatic and not progress to the clinical stage [3].

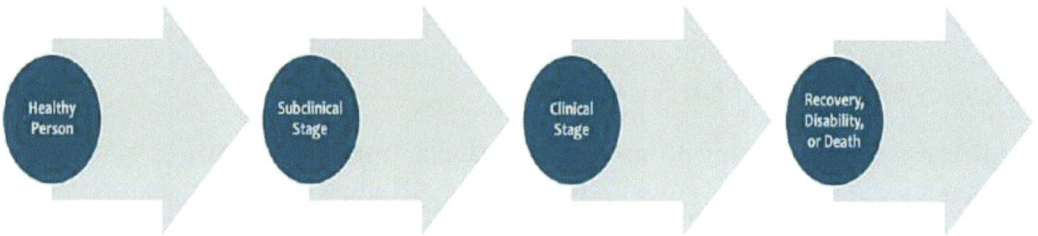

Fig. (3). Spectrum of disease.

For an infectious agent to cause infection in a susceptible person, there has to be an interplay between the amount of infective dose, virulence, and pathogenicity of the microbe. The challenge that public health practitioners face is that infected cases with mild or no symptoms and those incubated (carriers) often transmit the infection in the community. Similarly, although some people recover from a clinical infectious disease but remain infectious (*e.g.*, typhoid and hepatitis B infections), this class of people also ends up spreading the infection as healthy carriers. Thus, carriers could be – healthy, asymptomatic, passive, incubatory, or convalescent [3, 16].

Stages of Disease Progression

Understanding the natural history of a disease is vital for epidemiologists and healthcare professionals. The natural history outlines the typical progression of a disease from its initial onset to its resolution or chronicity. It helps identify key stages in disease development and provides insights into prevention and intervention opportunities [17]. The typical stages include:

1. Stage of Susceptibility: At this stage, individuals are susceptible to the disease but have not yet been exposed to the causative agent. Preventive measures, such as vaccination and health education, are essential to reduce susceptibility.

2. Stage of Exposure: Individuals are exposed to the causative agent, but they may not necessarily develop the disease. Monitoring and reducing exposure are key strategies at this stage.

3. Stage of Subclinical Disease: Some individuals develop subclinical or asymptomatic infections, meaning they carry the pathogen but do not show clinical signs. Surveillance and early detection efforts are critical to identify subclinical cases.

4. Stage of Clinical Disease: Individuals in this stage exhibit clinical symptoms and seek medical care. Early diagnosis, treatment, and isolation measures are essential to prevent further transmission.

5. Stage of Recovery, Disability, or Death: Depending on the disease, individuals may recover, experience disability, or succumb to the illness. Rehabilitation, supportive care, and end-of-life care are relevant interventions.

Prevention and Intervention Opportunities

The natural history of the disease provides valuable insights into when and where interventions can be most effective. Prevention and intervention strategies vary based on the disease stage, which are as follows [18]:

1. Primary Prevention: This focuses on reducing susceptibility and exposure. Examples include vaccination campaigns, health education, and environmental modifications to reduce exposure.

2. Secondary Prevention: At the stage of subclinical disease, secondary prevention aims to identify cases early and prevent clinical progression. Screening, diagnostic tests, and early treatment are key components.

3. Tertiary Prevention: For individuals with clinical disease, tertiary prevention focuses on reducing complications and disability and preventing death. It includes medical treatment, rehabilitation, and supportive care.

In understanding prevention and intervention opportunities, the reader needs to be familiar with the following terms [10 - 13, 18, 19]:

Epidemic is the increase in cases, usually as a result of the spread of the causative agent to what is considered normal in a population in a geographical area (*e.g.*, meningococcal meningitis with an attack rate of more than 15 cases per 100,000 for more than two weeks).

Endemic is the widespread constant presence of a disease in a geographic area (*e.g.*, malaria in sub-Saharan Africa).

Outbreak is the definition of an epidemic but in a limited geographic location. However, a reported case of a rare disease could be considered an outbreak (*e.g.*, polio, rabies, plague, *etc.*).

Hyperendemic is the persistently high levels of a disease in a geographical area (*e.g.*, dengue fever, malaria, *etc.*).

Holoendemic is when virtually everyone is infected (*e.g.*, malaria in some sub-Saharan countries).

Pandemic is an epidemic disease that has affected a large number of people and with global spread to several countries or continents (*e.g.*, COVID-19).

Sporadic cases are disease cases that infrequently occur in a given population (*e.g.*, gastroenteritis).

Cluster cases are the aggregation of cases in place and time above an otherwise expected number.

Exercise 3: Designing Interventions for Health Challenges

In this exercise, readers will apply their knowledge of the natural history of the disease to design interventions for specific health challenges:

i. **Select a Health Challenge**: Choose a health challenge or disease relevant to your community or region. Consider factors, such as disease prevalence, severity, and public health impact.
ii. **Map of the Natural History**: Analyze the natural history of the chosen health challenge. Identify the stages of disease progression and the typical outcomes at each stage.
iii. **Identify Intervention Points:** Determine the points along the natural history where interventions can be most effective. Consider primary, secondary, and tertiary prevention strategies.
iv. **Design Interventions:** Develop a comprehensive plan for intervention at each stage. Specify the activities, resources, and stakeholders involved in implementing the interventions.
v. **Evaluate Impact**: Discuss how these interventions could impact the health challenge. Consider potential barriers and challenges in implementing the interventions.

NB: This exercise empowers readers to apply their understanding of the natural history of the disease to real-world health challenges. It encourages critical thinking and the development of practical strategies for disease prevention and control.

EPIDEMIOLOGICAL FRAMEWORKS

Ecological and Multilevel Approaches

Epidemiological frameworks play a crucial role in understanding the complex interplay of factors that influence health outcomes. Two important frameworks often employed in epidemiology are ecological and multilevel approaches [20].

1. *Ecological Approach:* This approach considers the broader context in which individuals live, work, and interact. It examines the influence of environmental, social, and cultural factors on health outcomes. An ecological perspective recognizes that health is shaped not only by individual behaviours but also by community and societal factors. For example, studying the impact of air pollution on respiratory health at a neighbourhood level is an ecological approach.

2. *Multilevel Approach:* This approach recognizes that health determinants operate at multiple levels, including individual, interpersonal, community, and societal levels. It explores how factors at each level contribute to health disparities and outcomes. Multilevel analysis allows epidemiologists to investigate the relative importance of different factors and their interactions. For instance, studying how both individual-level factors (*e.g.*, smoking) and community-level factors (*e.g.*, access to healthcare) affect cancer rates is a multilevel approach.

Social Determinants of Health

Social Determinants of Health (SDOH) are the conditions in which people are born, grow, live, work, and age, and how these conditions can influence health outcomes. These determinants are critical factors that shape the overall well-being of an individual and are often more significant predictors of health outcomes than access to healthcare services alone. Social Determinants of health play a crucial role in shaping the health outcomes and health disparities of an individual more than individual behaviours. Addressing these determinants requires a holistic approach that combines policy change, community engagement, and healthcare interventions. By acknowledging and mitigating the impact of SDOH, we can work towards achieving health equity and improving the overall well-being of populations [21].

These determinants encompass a wide range of factors, including socioeconomic status, education, employment, housing, and access to healthcare. Epidemiologists often use social determinants of health as a framework to explore health disparities and inequities.

In this in-depth exploration of SDOH, we will examine various aspects, their impact on health, and strategies to address them.

Economic Stability

i. Income and employment are key components of economic stability. People with low incomes often face barriers to accessing essential resources, such as nutritious food, safe housing, and education.
ii. Poverty and unemployment can lead to chronic stress, inadequate housing, and reduced access to health care, all of which can negatively impact health.

Education:

i. Education level is strongly linked to health outcomes. Higher education is associated with better health, as it leads to better job opportunities, income, and access to healthcare.
ii. Lack of education can limit an individual's understanding of health information and their ability to make informed decisions about their well-being.

Neighbourhood and Physical Environment:

i. Living in safe, clean neighbourhoods with access to parks, grocery stores, and healthcare facilities positively impacts health.
ii. Conversely, living in environments with high crime rates, pollution, and limited access to fresh food can lead to chronic stress and increased risk of chronic diseases.

Social and Community Context:

i. Strong social support networks can provide emotional and practical assistance during times of need, promoting mental and physical health.
ii. Social isolation and discrimination can lead to mental health problems, substance abuse, and other adverse health outcomes.

Healthcare Access and Quality:

i. While access to healthcare is a determinant, it is also influenced by other SDOHS. Income, education, and neighbourhood conditions can affect one's ability to access and utilize healthcare services.
ii. Disparities in healthcare quality and availability further exacerbate health inequities.

Health Behaviors:

i. Lifestyle choices, such as diet, exercise, and substance use, are influenced by SDOH. For example, individuals in food deserts may have limited access to fresh, healthy foods.
ii. Education and income levels can also impact the ability of an individual to make healthier choices.

Social Determinants Across the Lifespan:

i. SDOH have lifelong effects on health. Early childhood experiences, like exposure to violence or malnutrition, can have lasting impacts on physical and mental health.
ii. Ageing populations face unique SDOH challenges, including access to social services and healthcare.

Addressing Social Determinants of Health:

Policymakers, healthcare providers, and communities can take the following steps to address SDOH:

1. Implement policies that reduce income inequality and poverty.

2. Invest in education, especially in underserved communities.

3. Create safe, walkable neighbourhoods with access to healthy food options.

4. Promote social cohesion and community engagement.

5. Expand access to healthcare services, especially in marginalized areas.

Exercise 4: Analyzing Social Determinants of Health in your Context

In this exercise, readers will analyze the social determinants of health in their local context to gain insights into health disparities and potential intervention points:

i. **Select a Health Issue:** Choose a specific health issue or condition that is relevant to your community or region. Consider diseases or health challenges with known disparities.
ii. **Identify Social Determinants:** Identify and list the key social determinants of health that are relevant to the chosen health issue. These may include factors, such as income, education, employment, housing, and access to healthcare.

iii. **Collect Data**: Gather data or information related to each identified social determinant. This can involve reviewing existing data, conducting surveys, or consulting local resources.

iv. **Analyze Disparities:** Analyze the data to determine if there are disparities in health outcomes based on different levels of social determinants. For example, assess whether individuals with lower income have higher rates of health issues compared to those with higher income.

v. **Identify Intervention Points:** Based on the analysis, we identify potential intervention points to address health disparities. Consider policies, programs, or initiatives that can target the social determinants identified.

vi. **Propose Interventions**: Develop a set of proposed interventions or recommendations to address the identified disparities. Describe how each intervention can impact the social determinants of health and improve health outcomes.

NB: This exercise empowers readers to apply the social determinants of the health framework to their local context. It encourages critical thinking about the factors that contribute to health disparities and the development of evidence-based interventions to promote health equity.

CONCLUSION

In conclusion, Chapter 2 has provided a comprehensive overview of epidemiological models and frameworks essential for understanding disease dynamics. By examining concepts, such as the Epidemiologic Triad, the chain of infection, and the natural history of the disease, readers have gained valuable insights into the multifaceted nature of epidemiological analysis. Furthermore, the exploration of various frameworks has equipped readers with diverse conceptual tools for interpreting and contextualizing epidemiological data. As readers delve deeper into subsequent chapters, they will continue to build upon these foundational models and frameworks, enriching their understanding of epidemiological principles and their applications in public health practice.

REFERENCES

[1]   Rothman KJ. Causes. Am J Epidemiol 1976; 104(6): 587-92.
        [http://dx.doi.org/10.1093/oxfordjournals.aje.a112335] [PMID: 998606]

[2]   Last JM. A dictionary of epidemiology. Oxford University Press 2001.

[3]   CDC. An Introduction to Applied Epidemiology and Biostatistics.Principles of Epidemiology in Public Health Practice. 3rd ed. Atlanta, GA: Centers for Disease Control and Prevention 2012; p. 30333.

[4]   Rothman KJ, Greenland S, Lash TL. Modern epidemiology. Lippincott Williams & Wilkins 2008.

[5]   CDC Principles of Epidemiology in Public Health Practice. Centers for Disease Control and Prevention 2021.

[6]   Royal College of Nursing. Chain of Infection. 2016. Available from: https://rcni.com/hosted-content/rcn/first-steps/chain-of-infection

[7]   Heymann DL. Control of Communicable Diseases Manual. American Public Health Association 2015.
        [http://dx.doi.org/10.2105/CCDM.2745]

[8]   John TJ, Samuel R. Herd immunity and herd effect: new insights and definitions. Eur J Epidemiol. 2000; 16(7): 601-6.
        [http://dx.doi.org/10.1023/A:1007626510002]

[9]   Natural History of Diseases: Statistical Designs and Issues. Clin Pharmacol Ther; 2016; 100(4): 353–361.
        [http://dx.doi.org/10.1002/cpt.423]

[10]   WHO. Emergencies. Disease outbreaks. 2020. Available from: https://www.who.int/emergencies/diseases/en/

[11]   CDC. Malaria. 2019. Retrieved from: https://www.cdc.gov/malaria/about/disease.html

[12]   WHO. Cholera. 2019. Available from: https://www.who.int/news-room/fact-sheets/detail/cholera

[13]   CDC. Coronavirus Disease 2019. Interim Clinical Guidance for Management of Patients with Confirmed Coronavirus Disease (COVID-19). 2020. Available from: https://www.cdc.gov/coronavirus/2019-ncov/hcp/clinical-guidance-management-patients.html

[14]   Galli SJ, Tsai M, Piliponsky AM. The development of allergic inflammation. Nature. 2008; 454(7203): 445–454.
        [http://dx.doi.org/10.1038/nature07204]

[15]   Bosman A. Incubation period, Latent period and Generation time. European Centre for Disease Prevention and Control. 2012; (5).

[16]   Helen C, Leggett HC, Cornwallis CK, West SA. Mechanisms of Pathogenesis, Infective Dose and Virulence in Human Parasites. PLoS Pathog. 2012; 8(2): e1002512.
        [http://dx.doi.org/10.1371/journal.ppat.1002512]

[17]   Kuller LH, Stoltzfus J. Epidemiology: concepts and applications. Oxford University Press 1989.

[18]   Koopman JS. The epidemic threshold of HIV transmission. AIDS 1989; 3(9): 661-7.

[19]   Principles of Epidemiology. 3rd ed. Atlanta, Georgia: Centers for Disease Control and Prevention 2012; p. 12.

[20]   Diez Roux AV. Investigating neighborhood and area effects on health. Am J Public Health 2001; 91(11): 1783-9.
        [http://dx.doi.org/10.2105/AJPH.91.11.1783] [PMID: 11684601]

[21]   Solar O, Irwin A. A conceptual framework for action on the social determinants of health. Social Determinants of Health Discussion Paper 2 (Policy and Practice). World Health Organization. 2010

CHAPTER 3

Epidemiological Research Design

Abstract: Chapter 3 provides an in-depth exploration of the fundamental components and methodologies involved in conducting epidemiological research. Beginning with an introduction to the themes of the chapter, it delves into research paradigms and study types prevalent in epidemiology. The chapter offers practical guidance on conducting epidemiological investigations, from study design to data collection and analysis. Moreover, it examines the statistical tools essential for rigorous epidemiological analysis, empowering readers with the skills needed to critically evaluate research findings and contribute to the advancement of public health knowledge.

Keywords: Data analysis, Epidemiological investigations, Epidemiological research Design, Research paradigms, Study types, Statistical tools.

INTRODUCTION

In our quest to decipher the mysteries of infectious diseases and their impact on human populations, we have embarked on a journey through the annals of epidemiology, exploring its history and the intricate web of models that underpin our understanding. In Chapter 3, the attention is to the foundation upon which epidemiology is built: research design.

Epidemiological research design is the compass that guides us through the uncharted territory of data collection, analysis, and interpretation. It is the blueprint that ensures our investigations are rigorous, methodical, and capable of providing insights that stand up to scrutiny. In this chapter, the focus is on the art and the science of designing epidemiological studies, where every decision, from selecting study populations to measuring outcomes carries profound implications for the knowledge we seek to uncover.

The exploration begins with a fundamental question: How do we design studies that allow us to investigate the intricate tapestry of disease transmission and its determinants? The answer lies in the careful selection of study designs tailored to the unique characteristics of the research question at hand. Whether it's a cross-sectional survey to capture a snapshot of disease prevalence, a cohort study tracking the health trajectories of individuals over time, or a case-control study seeking to identify risk factors, each design carries its own strengths and limitations.

As we journey deeper into this chapter, we will unravel the intricacies of epidemiological research design. We will explore the principles of randomization and blinding, discuss the importance of sample size and statistical power, and navigate the treacherous waters of confounding and bias, which can distort our findings if left unchecked. Through examples and case studies, we will witness how the choice of study design can profoundly influence the validity and generalizability of our results.

But epidemiological research design is not confined to the drawing board; it extends into the field, where data is collected, and laboratories, where analyses are conducted. We will also explore the practical aspects of data collection, from survey instruments and questionnaires to the ethical considerations that underpin human subject research. Additionally, we will delve into the nuances of data management and statistical techniques that enable us to extract meaningful insights from the vast troves of information we gather.

In the era of big data and technological innovation, epidemiological research design is undergoing a revolution. The integration of genomics, digital health records, and real-time surveillance systems has opened new frontiers in our ability to track and understand disease dynamics. In this chapter, we will glimpse into the future of epidemiological research, where interdisciplinary collaboration and cutting-edge technologies are reshaping the landscape of disease investigation.

As we embark on this chapter's journey into the realm of Epidemiological Research Design, remember that the quality of our research design determines the quality of our insights. It is the key that unlocks the doors to knowledge, enabling us to confront infectious diseases with precision and foresight. Welcome to Chapter 3, where we explore the art and science of designing epidemiological studies, paving the way for a deeper understanding of the complex interactions that govern the spread of diseases in our world.

RESEARCH PARADIGMS IN EPIDEMIOLOGY

As we know, different disciplines have different paradigms, and epidemiology is no exception. The purpose of the paradigm of research is to help us define how the world works, how knowledge is extracted from this world, and how a person thinks, writes, and talks about this knowledge. As popularised by Thomas Kuhn, the design is shaped by the models or belief systems we use to organise our reasoning and observations when conducting research [1].

A *paradigm*, a set of assumptions and perceptual orientations conceptualised by a community of researchers, determines how research communities view the phenomena they study and the methods to adopt in studying those phenomena [2]. In a scholarly context, there is a shared belief that science is not limited to specific epistemological or methodological criteria but to generate knowledge that improves life. Similarly, epidemiology has undoubtedly contributed immensely to identifying various disease risk factors and promoting population health, hence the growing call for participatory research to help bridge the gap between description and action [3].

People view social reality differently in natural and social sciences, which may limit their thinking and reasoning about the phenomenon in question. When solving social problems, a group of *conservatives* and *liberals* would have different views or perceptions on the role of government in addressing a social issue. Thus, how we view the world and structure our thoughts differs because our paradigms differ. For example, a *conservative* may believe that privatising healthcare is the best way to improve healthcare services. At the same time, a *liberal* would believe that the best way to address this is by employing more doctors in health services [1].

The three most common paradigms in the social sciences are *positivism, constructivism (or interpretivism), and pragmatism.*

1. Positivism, equated with quantitative research methods, is a doctrine by French philosopher Auguste Comte (1798–1857) and is considered a mixture of rationalism and empiricism. He suggested that the theory and observations are interdependent. He added that while reasoning is used in creating theories, they become authentic only if they are verified through observations [4]. In the early 20th century, the *antipositivists,* who belonged to the German idealism school of thought and equated with qualitative research methods, rejected the strong accounts of the positivists. Antipositivists are sometimes called interpretive sociologists because they emphasise that social actions must be studied through interpretive means [5].

2. Constructivism opines that researchers should reflect upon the paradigms that underpin their research. Thomas Kuhn argued that changes in how scientists view actual results from group dynamics and not only the subjective elements [1]. Constructivists, who oppose the philosophy of objectivism (rational individualism), believe in the existence of normative dimensions. They embrace the belief that humans can come to know the truth about the natural world without considering scientific approximations regarding validity and accuracy [6, 7].

3. Pragmatism is a philosophical doctrine that includes people who argue that an ideology or proposition is to be considered true as long as it works satisfactorily. This doctrine is a distinctly an American philosophical tradition and advocates accepting practical ideas and rejecting unpractical ones. An example of this is to address problems logically and practically [8].

Philosophically speaking, the paradigms are further examined based on the following three main pillars [9].

- *Ontology:* How we see the world; how we experience reality. The argument about whether the world consists of social order or constant change.
- *Epistemology:* How we acquire and process knowledge; our assumptions on how best to study the universe. The argument on whether we should use an objective or subjective approach to explore social reality.
- *Methodology:* How we design our studies to understand the universe. It is the systematic theoretical analysis of the research methods, which can be obtained through quantitative (deductive theory-testing), qualitative (inductive theory-building), or mixed approaches.

Thus, a psychologist, an epidemiologist, an anthropologist, and an economist interact with the world and define knowledge differently. Arguably, in its quest to answer research questions about individuals or groups, locally or globally, epidemiological studies require a quantitative approach (*e.g.*, statistical data) and qualitative (*e.g.* narrative). However, the approach to synthesise data may differ depending on the underlying research paradigm (*e.g.*, positivism in experimental design or constructivism in interpretative design). In epidemiological studies, data collection and analyses, measurable in the strictest sense, have standard statistical and modelling tools to test the strength of the relationships between the variables studied [10]. In this discussion, and within the research paradigm, epidemiology is characterised by a positivist standpoint.

Epidemiological Research

Epidemiological research plays a crucial role in understanding the causes and patterns of diseases within populations. Epidemiological research can be broadly categorized into two main paradigms: observational and experimental [11].

- *Observational Studies:* Observational studies are non-interventional investigations where researchers observe and collect participant data without intervening or manipulating variables. These studies are valuable for exploring associations, risk factors, and natural history of diseases. Common types of observational studies include cross-sectional, cohort, and case-control studies.

• *Experimental Studies:* Experimental studies, on the other hand, involve the deliberate manipulation of one or more variables to determine their effect on an outcome. These studies can establish cause-and-effect relationships. Randomized controlled trials (RCTs) are the gold standard for experimental studies in epidemiology, as they provide a high level of control over confounding variables and allow for causal inference.

When conducting epidemiological studies, it is necessary to choose the appropriate design and factors in their strengths and weaknesses, sources of bias, and confounders. It encompasses various study designs, including observational and experimental studies, each with its unique characteristics and purposes [11]. Additionally, study design considerations are essential to ensure the validity and reliability of research findings.

The choice between observational and experimental study design depends on the research question, feasibility, ethical considerations, and the level of control needed. Regardless of the study design, careful planning, attention to study design considerations, and understanding the various epidemiological studies are essential for producing meaningful and reliable results in epidemiology. Each study design has its strengths and limitations, and researchers should select the most appropriate approach based on their research objectives and constraints. Let us explore the interlink between these concepts and different types of epidemiological studies, including cross-sectional, cohort, case-control, and intervention studies [11].

In the design stage, and to effectively interpret the data, researchers must have a clear case definition of the symptoms and signs of the disease being investigated. Similarly, they must be able to define who is an exposed person, who is a probable case, and who is a confirmed case. Similarly, ethical considerations must be observed as with any form of research [12].

Study Design Considerations

Choosing the appropriate study design is crucial in epidemiological research. Several factors should be considered when selecting a study design [13]:

1. Research Question: The research question or hypothesis guides the choice of study design. For example, if the goal is to investigate the association between smoking and lung cancer, a cohort study or case-control study may be appropriate.

2. Availability of Data: Consider the availability of existing data and resources. Some study designs require extensive data collection and may be more resource-intensive.

3. Temporal Relationship: Determine whether the study aims to assess the temporal relationship between exposure and outcome. Cohort studies are particularly suited for evaluating cause-and-effect relationships over time.

4. Ethical Considerations: Ethical considerations, such as the feasibility of randomization in experimental studies or the protection of human subjects' rights and the well-being of study participants, must be addressed.

5. Sample Size: An adequate sample size is essential to ensure the study's statistical power and the ability to detect meaningful associations or differences.

6. Validity and Reliability: Researchers must employ valid and reliable measurement and data collection techniques to ensure the quality of their results.

7. Bias and Confounding: Researchers must consider potential sources of bias and confounding and implement strategies to minimize them. Researchers must address selection bias, information bias, and confounding to ensure the accuracy of their findings. Proper study design and data collection methods can help mitigate these biases.

8. Follow-up and Retention: In longitudinal studies (*e.g.,* cohort studies), maintaining a high rate of follow-up and participant retention is essential to minimize attrition bias.

Exercise 1: Choosing Study Designs for Local Health Issues

In this exercise, readers will apply their understanding of observational and experimental study designs to choose appropriate designs for investigating local health issues:

- Select a Local Health Issue: Choose a specific health issue or research question that is relevant to your local community or region. Consider issues with significant health implications.
- Define the Research Question: Clearly define the research question related to the chosen health issue. For example, if investigating the impact of a community-based intervention on diabetes prevalence, the question might be: "Does the community intervention reduce diabetes prevalence among residents?"

- Consider Study Objectives: Determine the objectives of the study. Are you primarily interested in establishing causation, exploring associations, or assessing risk factors?
- Review Resources: Assess the availability of resources, data, and ethical considerations for conducting the study. Consider the feasibility of implementing experimental designs if needed.
- Choose a Study Design: Based on the research question, objectives, and available resources, choose an appropriate study design. Explain why you believe this design is the most suitable for addressing the research question.

This exercise encourages readers to think critically about study design choices and apply their knowledge to real-world health issues in their local context. It promotes the selection of study designs that align with research goals and available resources.

STUDY TYPES IN EPIDEMIOLOGY

Epidemiological research plays a crucial role in understanding the causes and patterns of diseases within populations and can be broadly categorized into two main paradigms: observational studies and experimental studies. When conducting epidemiological studies, it is necessary to choose the appropriate design and factors in their strengths and weaknesses, sources of bias, and confounders. It encompasses various study designs, including observational and experimental studies, each with its unique characteristics and purposes [14].

Additionally, study design considerations are essential to ensure the validity and reliability of research findings. The choice between observational and experimental study design depends on the research question, feasibility, ethical considerations, and the level of control needed. Regardless of the study design, careful planning, attention to study design considerations, and an understanding of the various epidemiological studies are essential for producing meaningful and reliable results in epidemiology [14].

Each study design has its strengths and limitations, and researchers should select the most appropriate approach based on their research objectives and constraints. Let us explore the interlink between these concepts and different types of epidemiological studies, including cross-sectional, cohort, case-control, and intervention studies. In the design stage, and to effectively interpret the data, researchers must have a clear case definition of the symptoms and signs of the disease being investigated [14]. Similarly, they must be able to define who is an exposed person, who is a probable case, and who is a confirmed case. Similarly, ethical considerations must be observed as with any form of research [12].

Observational Studies

In observational studies, researchers observe and collect data on individuals or populations without intervening or manipulating any variables. The researchers do not control anything but observe and measure, allowing nature to take its course. This approach allows for examining associations and relationships between variables but does not establish causation. Types of observational studies include cross-sectional, case-control, and cohort studies. As shown in Table **1**, there are two broad types of observational studies – descriptive (cross-sectional, ecological) and analytical (case-control, cohort) [15, 16]. The observations obtained from descriptive and analytical studies could be used in generating testable hypotheses to help better understand the risk factors and causality that guide decision-making. The measurement parameters used in epidemiological studies, which will be discussed in later chapters, are prevalence, incidence, and mortality [15 - 18].

Table 1. The types of epidemiological studies [13].

Type of Study	Unit of Analysis
Observational studies	
i. Descriptive studies	
a. Cross-sectional	Individuals
b. Ecological	Populations
ii. Analytical studies	
a. Case-control	Individuals
b. Cohort	Individuals
Experimental studies	
i. Randomized controlled trials	Individuals
ii. Field trials	Healthy people
iii. Community trials	Healthy people/communities
iv. Quasi	Individuals

- *Descriptive* studies identify patterns among cases in each population by time (when), place (where), and person (who); descriptive studies help to estimate the number of people affected by a disease within a given population using specific characteristics such as symptoms and signs. The outcome of descriptive studies produces credible and reliable data, which could be used to identify trends and guide decision-making. Examples of descriptive studies are cross-sectional and ecological studies [15 - 18].
- *Analytic* studies identify and quantify the relationship between two or more variables, *e.g.*, exposure and health outcome (what). In analytic studies, the key

feature here is the comparison arm; it looks for causes (why) and effects (how), helps quantify the associations between exposure and outcomes, and formulates hypotheses that test for causal relationships. The investigators always try to find if a person or persons with a certain characteristic (extrinsic or intrinsic) are more likely to contract a disease than those without the characteristic; that characteristic is then associated with the disease. The outcome of analytical studies helps institute control, preventive measures, and guidance in policy making. Examples of analytical studies are case-control and cohort studies [15 - 18].

- **Cross-sectional** studies enroll a cross-section of the populace to measure exposure and health outcomes. This approach is routinely deployed to estimate disease prevalence and health outcomes, which is why it is referred to as prevalence studies. In research, cross-sectional studies are easy, inexpensive to carry out, and easy to measure exposure and effect simultaneously. In the study design, the critical question is whether exposure precedes or follows the effect. However, if the exposure data represents exposure before effect, the data could be treated like data generated from a cohort study. It is vital to note that conducting cross-sectional surveys on a representative sample of the population helps in knowing disease frequency and risk factors about age, sex, and ethnicity [17 - 20].

- **Cohort** studies follow a group of individuals (the cohort) to examine the development of health outcomes over time. Researchers categorize participants based on exposure status and assess the incidence of outcomes. Cohort studies are excellent for evaluating causation and identifying risk factors. Cohort studies involve an exposed and unexposed group of individuals with the same attributes to compare the disease rates in the exposed and unexposed groups to understand better the risk factors for health outcomes (Fig. **1**) [15 - 18].

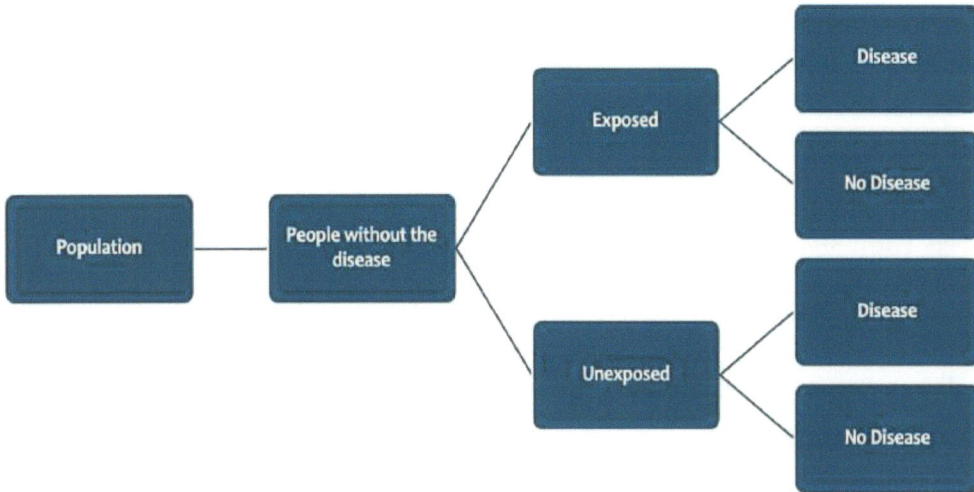

Fig. (1). The cohort study design.

Here, and unlike experimental studies, the investigator only observes and does not determine the exposure status of the participants. Cohort studies are sometimes referred to as *incidence* or *follow-up* studies because the follow-up time could be for a long period as the disease being studied may occur after a long time of exposure (*e.g.*, the effect of radiation on leukaemia or thyroid cancer as the time required for an outcome takes several years hence the need for follow up). However, sometimes difficulties do arise in tracking down individuals and with a resultant loss to follow-up after a time interval [17 - 19, 21].

One of the significant challenges in cohort studies is the *loss of follow-up,* which occurs when participants drop out of the study before its completion. This issue can introduce bias, particularly if the loss is related to the exposure or the outcome being studied [11,31,32].

If a substantial number of participants are lost, especially if the loss is differential (*e.g.*, more participants with higher risk are lost), the study's validity can be compromised. This can lead to underestimating or overestimating the association between exposure and outcome.

However, there are some strategies to mitigate loss to follow-up [11,31,32]. These strategies include:

- Regular communication with participants, providing incentives, and minimizing the burden of participation can help reduce dropouts.
- Data analysis adjustment techniques such as sensitivity analyses, imputation

methods, or statistical models that account for censored data (*e.g.*, survival analysis) can help mitigate the effects of loss to follow-up.

In contrast to cross-sectional studies, cohort studies are longitudinal, and the data is gathered over time for the same subjects over the study duration. The exposure could be for a brief (*e.g.*, retrospective as in a food poisoning outbreak) or more extended time (*e.g.*, prospective as in lung cancer or heart disease). In the context of risk ratio (*i.e.*, relative risk), the measure of the association between the risk factors and the disease would be known (see the example in Table **2**). The measure of association is an epidemiological measure that quantifies the relationships between exposure and a health event; the commonest are risk ratio, attributable risk, and odds ratio. The types of cohort studies include:

- *Prospective:* participants are followed over time to monitor them for disease occurrence
- *Retrospective:* participants are asked about their history retrospectively
- *Retrospective-prospective:* participants are asked about their history retrospectively and then followed prospectively for a disease of interest.

Using the two-by-two table (Table 2.2), Risk Ratio (RR) =

Incidence in the exposed (A/A+B) / Incidence in the unexposed (C/C+D).

If RR = 1.0, there is no difference in the risk between the exposed and unexposed groups

If RR is > 1.0, there is an increased risk for the exposed group.

If RR is < 1.0, there is a reduced risk for the exposed group.

Example 1: In 2015, there was a reported suspected measles outbreak in a rural area in Nigeria. As shown in Table **2**, out of the samples taken for testing, 2 out of the 114 children vaccinated against measles turned out to be positive for measles compared with 45 out of 60 unvaccinated children. Calculate the risk ratio.

Table 2. Example of two-by-two table.

	Ill	Not Ill	Total
Vaccinated	A (2)	B (112)	A+B (114)
Unvaccinated	C (45)	D (15)	C+D (60)
Total	A+C (47)	B+D (127)	A+B+C+D (174)

Risk of measles among vaccinated children = 2/114 = 0.0175 = 1.75%
Risk of measles among unvaccinated children = 45/60 = 0.75 = 75%
The RR = 0.0175/0.75 = 0.023

While extensive cohort studies are often costly, this can be reduced by using historical cohorts using records of previous exposure or registers of nurses, medical doctors, military personnel, twins, *etc.*, as these records routinely form part of the follow-up. Examples of cohort studies include evaluating the health effects of oral contraceptive use, associating Helicobacter pylori with gastric cancer, the study of identical twins, where the confounding factor is genetic variation, the Framingham study that investigated the risk factors for a wide range of diseases and this include cardiovascular, respiratory, and musculoskeletal disorders [17 - 23].

- *Cross-sectional* studies enroll a cross-section of the populace to measure exposure and health outcomes. This approach is routinely deployed to estimate disease prevalence and health outcomes, and that is why it is referred to as *prevalence* studies. In research, cross-sectional studies are easy, inexpensive to carry out, and easy to measure exposure and effect at the same time. Cross-sectional studies involve collecting data from a sample of individuals at a single point in time. They help to assess the prevalence of a particular condition or risk factors within a population. They do not establish causation but provide valuable insights into associations. In the study design, the critical question to ask is whether exposure precedes or follows the effect. However, if the exposure data represents exposure before effect, the data could be treated like data generated from a cohort study. It is vital to note that conducting cross-sectional surveys on a representative sample of the population helps in knowing disease frequency and risk factors about age, sex, and ethnicity [17 - 23].

- *Case-control* studies involve cases (individuals with the disease) and controls (individuals without the disease). Here, researchers compare individuals with a specific health outcome (case) to those without the outcome (controls). The goal is to identify factors that may have contributed to the development of the condition. Case-control studies are particularly useful for rare diseases. This case-control study, which is often done when the route of exposure is unknown, is usually retrospective (Fig. **2**). Here, epidemiologists look at the data retrospectively to know if a particular outcome can be linked to a suspected risk factor to prevent recurrence [17 - 23].

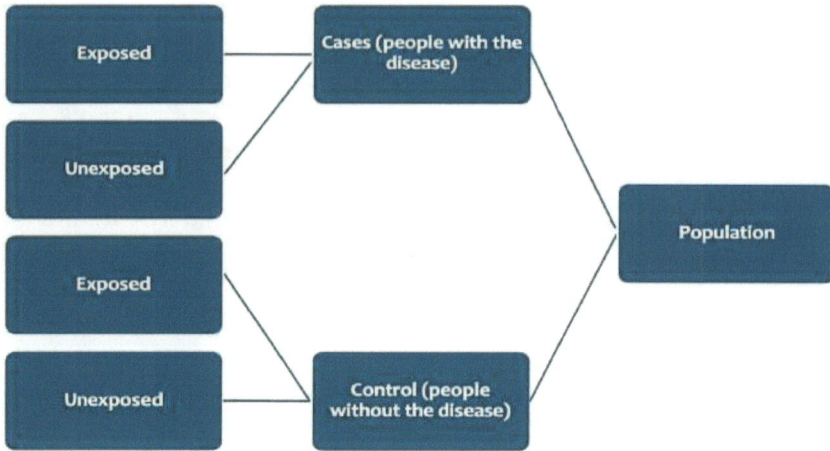

Fig. (2). The case-control study design.

In case-control studies, the investigators hypothesise the disease or outbreak's possible causes (risk factors). They then enroll a group of people with a disease (cases) and those without it (controls, comparison, or reference). While the selection is based on disease and not exposure, finding the most cost-effective way to identify and enroll control subjects is critical. Furthermore, note that accurate timing of exposure to an agent (*e.g.*, a drug) is sometimes crucial in determining the relevant exposure. As with cohort studies, case-control is longitudinal and can be retrospective or prospective depending on the situation of the disease under study.

An example of a retrospective case-control study is establishing the relationship between thalidomide use in the first trimester and limb defects in newborn babies. This study conducted in 1961 in Germany compared affected children with healthy children born between 1959-60. Out of the 46 mothers who gave birth to babies with limb malformations, 41 received treatment for hyperemesis gravidarum using thalidomide in the trimester. However, none of the 300 control mothers with healthy children had thalidomide during pregnancy [19].

Another typical example is a study examining a causal link between smoking and lung cancer.

Using Odds Ratio (OR), the measure of association for case-control studies would be known. Thus, using the two-by-two table,

OR = Odds that cases were exposed (AD) / Odds that cases were not exposed (BC).

Example: In a retrospective case-control study conducted in 1998 to look at the association between cigarette smoking and lung cancer in a Nigerian state, 112 out of 1,450 adult smokers developed lung cancer compared with 22 of the 1,525 adult non-smokers (Table **3**). Calculate the risk and odds ratio.

Table 3. Example of two-by-two table.

	Ill	Not Ill	Total
Exposed	A (112)	B (1,338)	A+B (1,450)
Unexposed	C (22)	D (1,503)	C+D (1,525)
Total	A+C (134)	B+D (2,841)	2,975

The risk of cancer of the lungs among smokers = 112/1450 = 7.724

The risk of cancer of the lungs among non-smokers = 22/1525 = 0.014

The Risk Ratio = 7.724/0.014 = 551.7

The OR = (112/1338) / (22/1503) = 112*1503/1338*22 = 168336 / 29436 = 5.72. This implies that the cases were 5.72 times more likely than the controls to have been exposed. The odds ratio and risk ratio are very similar, especially when dealing with a rare disease, hence the need to have a good representative of the general population concerning exposure. Case-control studies are sometimes referred to as case-reference studies and are useful in so many ways - helping to look into the factors that affect the health and illness of a given population, quickly and easily because it doesn't require waiting for months or years as it is usually based on past data, doesn't require large participants to be statistically significant, and ethical challenges are minimal. However, the limitations including data quality, recall bias, cause, and effect may not prove a link, sampling bias as cases and controls may not be truly representative, etc [17 - 23].

- *Ecological* studies, also referred to as correlational studies, use groups of people rather than individuals as units of analysis, and are useful in generating hypotheses. Ecological studies could be used to compare different populations in two or more countries at the same time, or to compare the same population in one place at different times; the latter is known as the time series. While ecological studies often rely on data collected for a different purpose, the outcome cannot link at the individual level between exposure and effect. There is a term 'ecological fallacy' or bias that occurs when there is a lack of relationship between two variables (*e.g.*, maternal deaths and the absence of skilled birth attendants in the region under study) [17, 18].

- *Intervention* studies, often referred to as experimental or clinical trials, involve the deliberate manipulation of a variable or the implementation of an intervention to assess its impact on health outcomes. Randomized controlled trials (RCTs) are a common type of intervention study.

Experimental Studies

In experimental studies, researchers manipulate who gets what or does what and then follow up with the subjects (clinical trial), field trial, or community (community trial) over time to determine the effects of an intervention by comparing the outcome of the exposure in both the experimental and control groups. The commonest example here is testing a new drug or vaccine on a selected group of patients or persons. However, ethical considerations (*e.g.*, participants have an equal right to get the drug, informed consent must be sought, and treatment must be safe for the participants) are critical; hence, there is a need for study protocols to address that at the study design stage [15]. As shown in Table **1**, experimental studies are divided into randomised controlled trials (RCT), field trials, community trials, and quasi-experiments [14, 17, 18, 24].

- *Randomised controlled trials:* Researchers randomly assign *patients* to intervention and control groups to assess the effects of a particular intervention (*e.g.*, drug or vaccine) on the disease under study and the outcomes compared [13, 14, 20, 21].
- *Field trials:* Researchers randomly assign *healthy people* in the general population presumed to be at risk of a specific disease to preventive intervention and control arms, follow up with the subjects, and measure the outcomes. Field trial studies can be on a smaller scale (*e.g.*, blood lead level measurements in children to protect them from lead poisoning in lead paint, at a lower cost and short follow-up) or larger (*e.g.*, Salk vaccine for the prevention of poliomyelitis) scale as the case may be [14, 17, 18, 24 - 26].
- *Community trials:* Researchers use communities rather than individuals as treatment groups to study the influence of social conditions on diseases and target group behaviour as prevention efforts. A good example here is cardiovascular disease. However, the lack of internal validity is a key limitation of this type of design (*e.g.*, random allocation of communities is not possible, accommodates only a small number of communities, *etc.*) [14, 17, 18, 24 - 26].
- *Quasi-experimental,* which means 'resembling', is not truly an experimental study. It estimates an intervention's causal impact or evaluates the treatment's effectiveness. In quasi-design, the independent variable is manipulated but without the random assignment of the participants to conditions or orders of conditions; this makes it between correlational studies and true experiments, thus raising concerns about internal validity. An example would be a drug trial

for hypertension, randomly assigning enrollees to a new antihypertensive, an existing antihypertensive drug, or lifestyle modification. The various types of quasi-studies include non-equivalent group designs, pretest-posttest, and interrupted time-series designs [14, 17, 18, 24 - 26].

Ethical Considerations

Epidemiological research must adhere to ethical principles to protect the rights and well-being of study participants and ensure the validity and credibility of findings [27]. Ethical considerations are paramount in epidemiological research, given the potential implications for public health and individual participants. Ethical principles guide the design, conduct, and reporting of research to ensure the protection of participants' rights and well-being. Key ethical considerations include [33,34,35]:

1. Informed Consent: Obtaining informed consent is a fundamental ethical requirement. Participants must provide informed and voluntary consent to participate in the study. Researchers should provide clear information about the study's purpose, procedures, risks, benefits, and their right to withdraw at any time without penalty. The process must ensure that participants understand the information provided and voluntarily agree to participate. Ensuring truly informed consent can be challenging in studies involving vulnerable populations or complex scientific concepts. Researchers must use clear and accessible language, and in some cases, provide additional support, such as translators or cultural mediators.

2. Privacy and Confidentiality: Protecting participants' privacy and ensuring the confidentiality of their data is paramount. Researchers must implement measures to secure personal data and ensure that participants' identities are not disclosed. This includes anonymizing data, using secure data storage systems, and restricting data access to authorized personnel only. A breach of confidentiality can lead to stigma, discrimination, or legal consequences for participants. It can also undermine public trust in research and deter future participation.

3. Beneficence and Non-Maleficence: Researchers must balance the potential risks and benefits of the study. Researchers must prioritize the well-being of participants and minimize potential harm. The principle of non-maleficence dictates that the research should not cause harm to participants, while the principle of beneficence requires that the study should aim to produce benefits that outweigh the risks. In some studies, particularly those involving experimental interventions, the risk-benefit balance can be difficult to ascertain. Ethical guidelines require assessing and mitigating the risks associated with the study.

Ethical review boards play a crucial role in evaluating these aspects before approving the study.

4. Justice and Equity: Ensure that research benefits are distributed fairly and that vulnerable populations are not exploited. Researchers should consider the potential impact of the study on various subgroups. The principle of justice requires that the benefits and burdens of research are distributed fairly. This means ensuring that no group is disproportionately burdened or excluded from the potential benefits of research.

Inclusion Criteria: Researchers should ensure that the study population reflects the diversity of the population affected by the health issue under investigation. This includes considering gender, race, socioeconomic status, and other relevant factors.

Avoiding Exploitation: Researchers must be vigilant to avoid exploiting vulnerable populations, such as those with limited access to healthcare or education, who might be unduly influenced to participate in research.

5. Ethical Oversight: All epidemiological research should undergo review by an independent ethics committee or institutional review board (IRB). This oversight ensures that the study adheres to ethical principles and that participants' rights and well-being are protected. Ethics committees should also oversee the study's progress, particularly in long-term cohort studies, to ensure that ethical standards are maintained throughout the research process.

Exercise 2: Addressing Ethical Dilemmas in Your Research

In this exercise, readers will grapple with ethical dilemmas commonly encountered in epidemiological research and explore strategies for addressing them:

- Select an Ethical Dilemma: Choose a hypothetical ethical dilemma related to epidemiological research. For example, you might consider a situation where obtaining informed consent is challenging or where the potential benefits of research may not be evenly distributed.
- Analyze the Dilemma: Describe the ethical dilemma in detail, considering the conflicting principles and potential consequences. Highlight the ethical principles involved, such as informed consent, privacy, and beneficence.
- Propose Ethical Solutions: Develop one or more ethical solutions or strategies for addressing the dilemma. Explain how each solution aligns with ethical principles and safeguards participants' rights and well-being.

- Consider Real-World Applications: Reflect on how your proposed solutions might be applied to actual epidemiological research in your local context. Discuss any challenges or considerations specific to your region.

This exercise encourages readers to think critically about the ethical dilemmas that may arise in their research endeavours and develop ethical solutions that uphold the principles of responsible and respectful research conduct. It promotes ethical awareness and decision-making in epidemiological research.

CONDUCTING EPIDEMIOLOGICAL INVESTIGATIONS

In investigating disease causation or association with a particular agent, epidemiologists try to study the health event rigorously to understand the concept fully. While applied epidemiology could be either a descriptive or an analytic approach, there is a need to use experience, epidemiologic insight, and a good understanding of the local conditions to arrive at a diagnosis and suggest realistic public health measures to control and or prevent a health event [17, 18]. Epidemiologists look at *'Who'* to know the person involved, *'What'* to establish a case definition, *'Where'* to see the setting or place of occurrence, *'When'* to understand the time the health event started, and *'Why'* to unravel the causes, risk factors, and mode of transmission. Let us explore the deeper meaning of these adverbs in the context of epidemiologic studies [17, 18].

Who: This counts the number of persons involved by converting case counts into risks or rates related to several cases to the size of the population. It is essential to take into consideration the intrinsic and extrinsic characteristics of the persons under study. The intrinsic (inherent) characteristics here include age, sex, and ethnic background. In contrast, the extrinsic (acquired) characteristics are immunity, SES such as education, housing, occupation, nutrition, health-related beliefs, behaviours (smoking, alcohol, health care seeking), *etc*. Epidemiologists present the analysed data in a tabular or graphical manner (Fig. **3**).

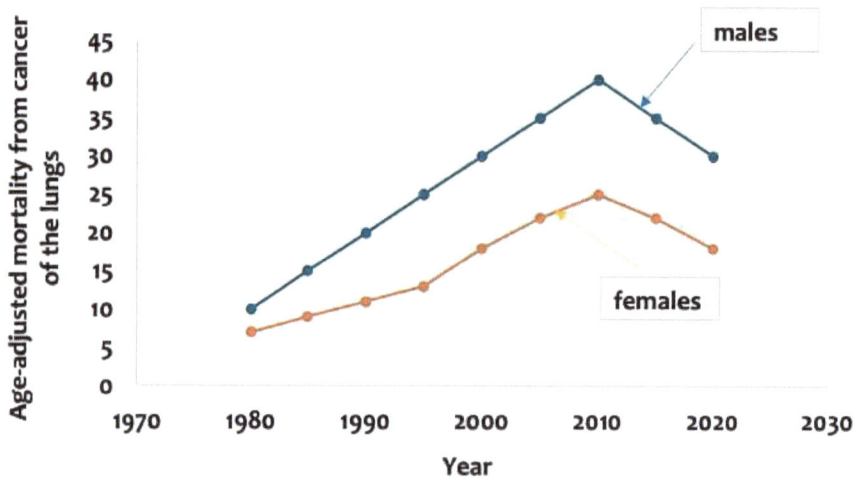

Fig. (3). An example of age-adjusted mortality from cancer of the lungs between males and females.

What: This question is all about case definition, which is a set of standard criteria used to establish whether a person does (or does not) have a disease or health-related events: symptoms, signs, or other supportive evidence, (+/- confirmatory lab results). However, this may sometimes have limitations on time, place & person.

Example: During the measles outbreak, a person may be classified based on the following: -

- Suspected: fever and rash.
- Probable: fever, rash, history of contact with a confirmed case.
- confirmed: fever, rash, positive serologic test for measles IgM ab.

Where: This question is about the place of the health event (*e.g.*, place of residence, place of work, hospital environment, district, state, or country). When the analysis is carried out based on the information obtained, then a clue would be obtained as to the source of the agent, mode of transmission, *etc*.

When: This question is about time, and we know that the rates of occurrence of the disease often change over time. Using this information to plot the annual rate of a disease over some time (years) helps to know the secular trend of the disease.

There are various ways of presenting information about a health event, either using a map (Fig. **4**) or a tabular form (Table **4**).

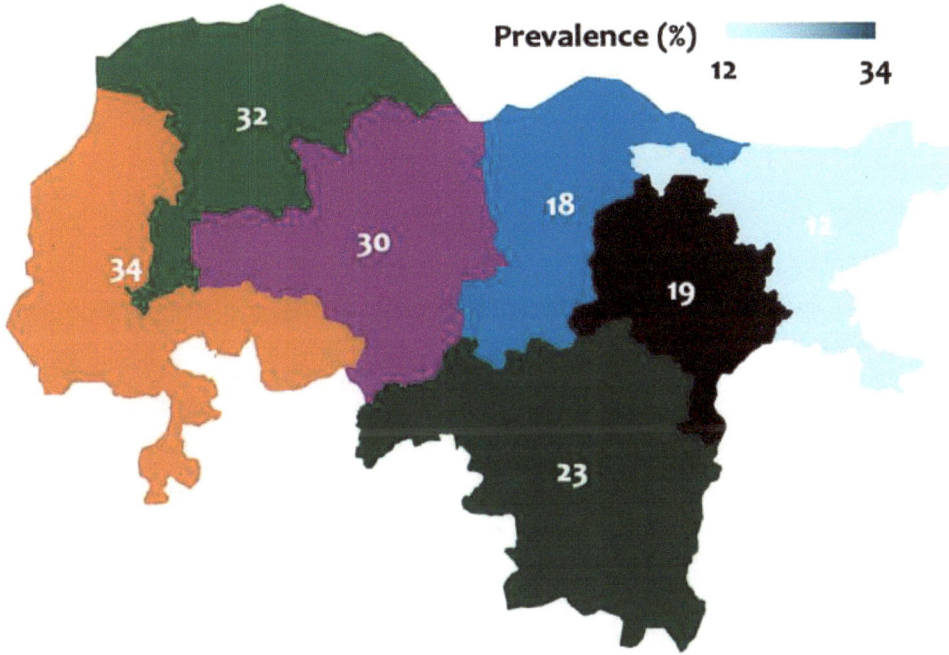

Fig. (4). An example showing a map of malaria prevalence in a survey conducted across states in country X.

Table 4. An example showing reported cases of COVID19 in a country X on 1st April 2020.

States	Total Reported Cases	Suspected Cases	Probable Cases	Total Confirmed Cases
A	20	15	4	1
B	8	4	2	2
C	13	10	2	1
D	23	18	3	2
E	8	6	2	0
Total	72	53	13	6

Other ways of presenting information include graphs of diseases; Fig. (**5**) shows the seasonality of a disease, Fig. (**6**) shows secular trends showing cases/rates over some time, and Fig. (**7**) shows the epi curve (epidemic curve) showing days over a period of time in outbreaks.

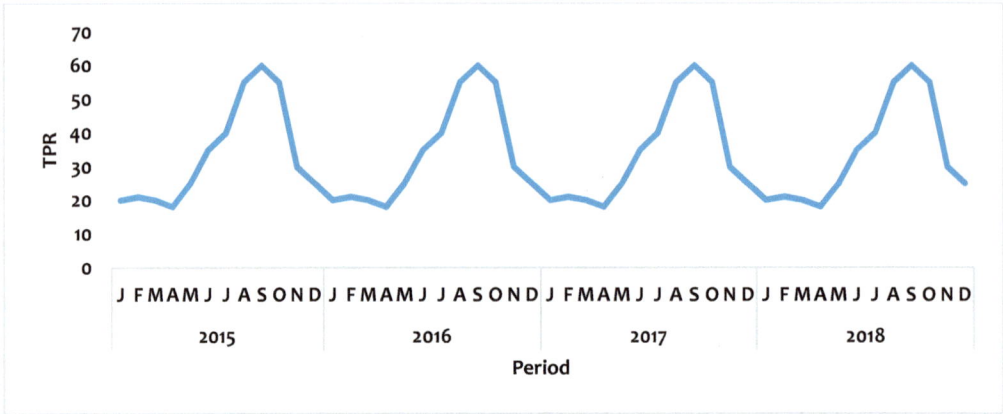

Fig. (5). An example of a line graph showing the seasonality of the malaria positivity rate (TPR) per 100,000 population.

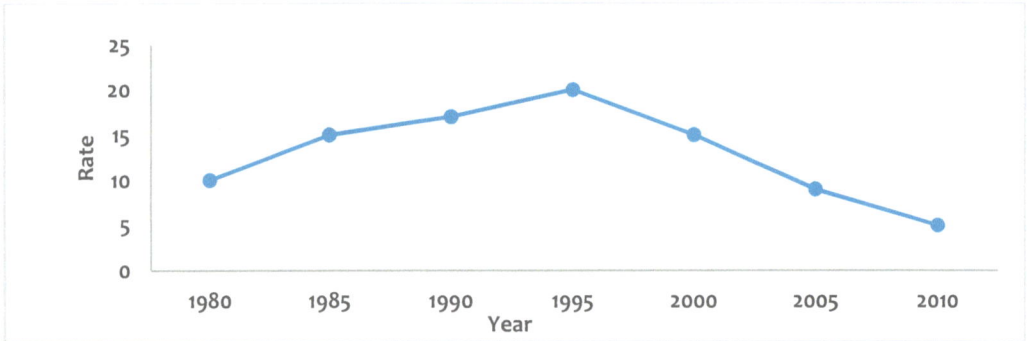

Fig. (6). A secular trends of Hepatitis A infection per 100,000 population, 1980 – 2010..

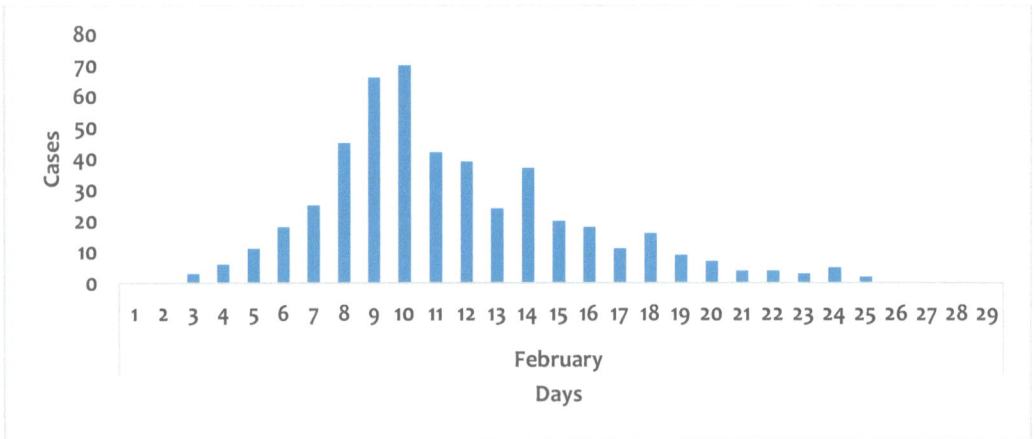

Fig. (7). An example of a bar chart of food poisoning outbreaks per 1,000 population.

Often, the shape of the epi curve guides epidemiologists to generate hypotheses about the source, time, transmission mode, and causative agent. Understanding, when diseases occur, does help in predicting the future incidence of disease and evaluating programmes or policy decisions.

Why: This question would help investigators to understand the causes. It tries to answer questions on the health event such as –

• Could the outbreak be due to a contaminated water source?
• Could it be due to the consumption of contaminated food?
• Could it be due to poor sanitary hygiene in a school?

The 'Why' is what analytic studies seek to answer; it helps to quantify the associations between exposure and outcomes and to formulate hypotheses that test for causal relationships.

Data Collection and Sampling Methods

Epidemiological investigations rely on the systematic collection and analysis of data to draw meaningful conclusions about health-related issues. The quality of the data collected and the appropriateness of sampling methods are critical to the validity and reliability of study findings [29].

Data Collection Methods

1. Surveys: Surveys are commonly used to gather information from study participants. Questionnaires and interviews are tools employed to collect data on health behaviours, symptoms, exposures, and other relevant variables.

2. Medical Records: For studies involving clinical data or patient information, medical records provide a valuable source of information. Researchers can extract data on diagnosis, treatment, and outcomes from patient records.

3. Biological Samples: Some epidemiological studies involve the collection of biological specimens such as blood, urine, or tissue samples. These samples can be analyzed for markers of disease, exposure, or genetic factors.

4. Environmental Monitoring: Environmental epidemiology often involves the collection of data on air quality, water quality, or other environmental factors that may impact health. Specialized monitoring equipment and sensors are used for data collection.

Sampling Methods

1. Random Sampling: Random sampling ensures that each member of the population has an equal chance of being included in the study. It minimizes selection bias and allows for the generalization of findings to the larger population.

2. Stratified Sampling: In stratified sampling, the population is divided into subgroups or strata, and random samples are drawn from each stratum. This method is useful when researchers want to ensure the representation of specific subgroups.

3. Convenience Sampling: Convenience sampling involves selecting participants based on their accessibility or convenience. While this method is less rigorous and may introduce bias, it can be practical for certain research questions.

Exercise 3: Collecting and Analyzing Local Health Data

In this exercise, readers will apply their knowledge of data collection and sampling methods to a practical scenario involving local health data:

- Select a Local Health Issue: Choose a specific health issue or topic relevant to your local community or region. This could be a prevalent disease, a health behaviour, or an environmental factor.
- Define Data Collection Objectives: Clearly, define the objectives of your data collection efforts. What specific information do you want to gather, and how will it contribute to addressing the chosen health issue?
- Choose Data Collection Methods: Based on your research objectives, select appropriate data collection methods. Consider whether surveys, medical records, biological samples, or environmental monitoring are the most relevant.
- Design a Sampling Strategy: Determine the target population for your data collection and design a sampling strategy. Will you use random sampling, stratified sampling, or another method? Explain your rationale.
- Collect and Analyze Data: If possible, carry out a mock data collection exercise in your local context. Analyze the data using basic statistical techniques or software tools. Summarize your findings and consider their implications for addressing the health issue.

This exercise provides hands-on experience in planning and conducting data collection for epidemiological investigations. It encourages readers to apply their knowledge to real-world health challenges and develop practical skills in data collection and analysis.

STATISTICAL TOOLS FOR EPIDEMIOLOGICAL ANALYSIS

Statistical tools for epidemiological analysis are a crucial field of study that combines statistics and epidemiology to analyze and understand patterns of diseases and health-related events within populations. *Epidemiology* is the science that investigates the distribution and determinants of health-related events in populations to improve public health. It plays a pivotal role in identifying the causes of diseases, evaluating interventions, and shaping health policies. Statistical tools and methods are the backbone of epidemiological analysis, enabling researchers to make sense of complex health data, draw meaningful conclusions, and make informed decisions [29]. The key concepts are:

1. Descriptive Epidemiology: Before diving into statistical analysis, epidemiologists often begin by describing the occurrence of a disease or health event in a population. This process involves calculating basic measures such as incidence rates, prevalence, and distribution by time, place, and person.

2. Inferential Statistics: Once the data is described, statistical tools infer relationships and associations. Standard statistical methods include hypothesis testing, regression analysis, and survival analysis. These techniques help researchers identify risk factors, assess causality, and make predictions.

3. Study Designs: Epidemiological studies can take various forms, including cohort studies, case-control studies, cross-sectional studies, and randomized controlled trials (RCTs). Each study design has statistical tools and analytical approaches to address specific research questions.

4. Bias and Confounding: In epidemiology, addressing bias and confounding is crucial. Bias refers to systematic errors in data collection or interpretation, while confounding occurs when an extraneous factor distorts the genuine relationship between an exposure and outcome. Statistical techniques are used to control for these sources of error.

5. Survival Analysis: Epidemiologists often analyze time-to-event data, such as the time until a disease develops or a person dies. Using tools like Kaplan-Meier curves and Cox proportional hazard models, survival analysis helps assess the influence of various factors on survival outcomes.

6. Spatial Analysis: Geography can play a significant role in disease distribution. Spatial statistics allow researchers to analyze geographic patterns of diseases and explore the spatial relationships between health outcomes and environmental factors.

*7. **Meta-analysis:*** Combining results from multiple studies through meta-analysis provides a more comprehensive view of the evidence and can yield more robust conclusions about the effects of interventions or exposures.

In the upcoming chapters, we will delve deeper into these concepts and discuss how statistical tools are applied in epidemiological research to uncover patterns, trends, and risk factors for various diseases. We will also explore real-world examples and case studies to illustrate the practical application of these statistical techniques in public health and epidemiology.

Descriptive and Analytic Statistics

Epidemiological analysis relies on statistical methods to summarize, interpret, and draw meaningful conclusions from data [29]. Two main categories of statistics are employed:

*1. **Descriptive Statistics*** are used to summarize and describe data. Common descriptive statistics include measures of central tendency (*e.g.*, mean, median, mode) and measures of variability (*e.g.*, range, variance, standard deviation). Descriptive statistics provide a snapshot of the data's characteristics.

*2. **Analytic Statistics***, also known as inferential statistics, are used to make inferences about a population based on a sample of data. Key concepts include hypothesis testing and confidence intervals. Researchers use these methods to assess associations, differences, and causality.

Hypothesis Testing and Inference

Hypothesis testing is a fundamental component of epidemiological analysis [30]. It involves the following steps:

*1. **Formulating Hypotheses:*** Researchers start by formulating a null hypothesis (H0) and an alternative hypothesis (H1). The null hypothesis typically represents no effect or no association, while the alternative hypothesis suggests an effect or association.

*2. **Data Collection and Analysis:*** Data is collected and analyzed using appropriate statistical tests. The choice of the test depends on the research question and the type of data (*e.g.*, categorical, continuous).

*3. **Calculating Test Statistics:*** Test statistics, such as t-tests, chi-square tests, or regression coefficients, are calculated to assess whether the observed differences or associations are statistically significant.

*4. **Setting Significance Levels:*** Researchers set a significance level (alpha) to determine the threshold for statistical significance. Common alpha values include 0.05 and 0.01. If the p-value (a measure of significance) is less than alpha, the results are considered statistically significant.

*5. **Interpreting Results:*** Based on the p-value and alpha, researchers decide whether to reject the null hypothesis or fail to reject it. Rejecting the null hypothesis suggests that there is a statistically significant effect or association.

Exercise 4: Analyzing Local Health Data Statistically

In this exercise, readers will practice applying statistical tools to analyze local health data:

- Select a Local Health Dataset: Obtain or access a dataset related to a local health issue or research question. This could be data on disease incidence, risk factors, or health outcomes.
- Define Research Questions: Clearly, define one or more research questions or hypotheses related to the dataset. For example, you might investigate whether there is a significant difference in disease rates between different age groups in your community.
- Choose the Appropriate Statistical Test: Based on your research questions and the type of data (categorical or continuous), select the appropriate statistical test (*e.g.*, t-test, chi-square test, regression analysis).
- Perform Statistical Analysis: Conduct the statistical analysis using software tools like Excel R, or specialized statistical software. Calculate relevant statistics, such as means, proportions, or odds ratios.
- Interpret the Results: Analyze the results of your statistical tests. Determine whether the observed differences or associations are statistically significant based on the chosen significance level (alpha).
- Draw Conclusions: Summarize your findings and draw conclusions based on the statistical analysis. Discuss the implications of your results for addressing the local health issue.

This exercise enables readers to gain practical experience in using statistical tools to analyze health data and make evidence-based decisions. It reinforces the importance of statistical rigour in epidemiological research and its impact on public health practice.

CONCLUSION

In conclusion, Chapter 3 has offered a comprehensive overview of epidemiological research design, encompassing key methodologies and statistical tools essential for conducting rigorous investigations. By exploring research paradigms, study types, and practical considerations in epidemiological research, readers have gained valuable insights into the intricacies of study design, data collection, and analysis. Moreover, the examination of statistical tools has equipped readers with the necessary skills to navigate complex datasets and derive meaningful conclusions. As readers progress through subsequent chapters, they will continue to build upon these foundational principles, further enhancing their proficiency in epidemiological research design and analysis.

REFERENCES

[1]　Kuhn TS. The Structure of Scientific Revolutions. Chicago: University of Chicago Press 1962.

[2]　Given LM. The SAGE encyclopedia of qualitative research methods. Thousand Oaks, CA: SAGE Publications, Inc. 2008; Vol. 1-0.
[http://dx.doi.org/10.4135/9781412963909]

[3]　Bach, M., Jordan, S., Hartung, S., Santos-Hövener, C., and Wright, M. T. 2017. Participatory epidemiology: the contribution of participatory research to epidemiology. Emerging themes in epidemiology, 14, 2. 2017.

[4]　Michel B. Auguste Comte The Stanford Encyclopedia of Philosophy (Summer 2018 Edition), Edward N. Zalta (ed.), URL = Available from:https://plato.stanford.edu/archives/sum2018/entries/comte/

[5]　Beiser, F.C. German Idealism: The Struggle Against Subjectivism, 1781-1801, Harvard University Press. 2002.

[6]　Crotty, M. The Foundations of Social Science Research: Meaning and Perspective in the Research Process, Sage. 1998.

[7]　Howell KE. Paradigm of Inquiry: Critical Theory and Constructivism. In: Howell K, Sorour M, Eds. Corporate Governance in Africa. London: Palgrave Macmillan 2016.
[http://dx.doi.org/10.1057/978-1-137-56700-0_2]

[8]　Legg, C. and Hookway, C. (2019). "Pragmatism", The Stanford Encyclopedia of Philosophy (Spring 2019 Edition), Edward N. Zalta (ed.), URL = Available from: https://plato.stanford.edu/archives/spr2019/entries/pragmatism/

[9]　Bhattacherjee, A. Social Science Research: Principles, Methods, and Practices. USF Open Access Textbooks Collection. 2012.

[10]　Bach M, Jordan S, Hartung S, Santos-Hövener C, Wright MT. Participatory epidemiology: the contribution of participatory research to epidemiology. Emerg Themes Epidemiol 2017; 14(1): 2.
[http://dx.doi.org/10.1186/s12982-017-0056-4] [PMID: 28203262]

[11]　Rothman, K. J., Greenland, S., & Lash, T. L.. Modern Epidemiology. Lippincott Williams & Wilkins. 2008.

[12]　Silman, A.J. and Macfarlane, G.J. Epidemiological Studies: A Practical Guide. Cambridge University Press, The Pitt Building, Trumpington Street, Cambridge, United Kingdom. 2002.

[13]　Szklo, M., & Nieto, F. J. Epidemiology: Beyond the Basics. Jones & Bartlett Learning. 2014.

[14]　Hennekens, C. H., & Buring, J. E. Epidemiology in Medicine. Little, Brown. 1987.

[15]   Kelsey, J.L., Whittemore, A.S, Evans, A.S, and Thompson, W.D. Methods in observational epidemiology. New York: Oxford University Press. 1996.

[16]   Kelsey, J.L. and Gold, E.B. Observational Epidemiology. In International Encyclopedia of Public Health, 2016 pp. 295-307.
[http://dx.doi.org/10.1016/B978-0-12-803678-5.00310-6]

[17]   Bonita, R., Beaglehole, R., and Kjellström T. Basic epidemiology 2nd ed. World Health Organ 2006.

[18]   CDC. An Introduction to Applied Epidemiology and Biostatistics. In Principles of Epidemiology in Public Health Practice. 3rd ed. Centers for Disease Control and Prevention, Atlanta, GA 30333. 2012.

[19]   Rothman, KJ., Greenland, S. and Lash, TL.Principles of Epidemiology. Key Concepts in Public Health. London: Sage UK. 2009.

[20]   Saleh JEA, Saddiq A, Adamu HI, Mpazanje R, Audu BM. Suspected Malaria Outbreak Investigations in Baure LGA, Katsina State, Nigeria. OAlib 2019; 6(7): 1-7.
[http://dx.doi.org/10.4236/oalib.1105512]

[21]   Guest, G. and Namey, E.E. Public Health Research Methods. SAGE Publications, Inc. 2014.

[22]   Vandenbroucke JP. Prospective or retrospective: what's in a name? BMJ 1991; 302(6771): 249-50.
[http://dx.doi.org/10.1136/bmj.302.6771.249] [PMID: 1998787]

[23]   Pearce N, Checkoway H. Cohort Studies. In: Melnick EL, Everitt BS, Eds. Encyclopedia of Quantitative Risk Analysis and Assessment. 2008.
[http://dx.doi.org/10.1002/9780470061596.risk0598]

[24]   Fortmann SP, Flora JA, Winkleby MA, Schooler C, Taylor CB, Farquhar JW. Community intervention trials: reflections on the Stanford Five-City Project Experience. Am J Epidemiol 1995; 142(6): 576-86.
[http://dx.doi.org/10.1093/oxfordjournals.aje.a117678] [PMID: 7653465]

[25]   Susser M. The tribulations of trials--intervention in communities. Am J Public Health 1995; 85(2): 156-8.
[http://dx.doi.org/10.2105/AJPH.85.2.156] [PMID: 7856769]

[26]   Shargie EB, Mørkve O, Lindtjørn B. Tuberculosis case-finding through a village outreach programme in a rural setting in southern Ethiopia: community randomized trial. Bull World Health Organ 2006; 84(2): 112-9.
[http://dx.doi.org/10.2471/BLT.05.024489] [PMID: 16501728]

[27]   Coughlin, S. S., & Beauchamp, T. L. Ethics and Epidemiology. Oxford University Press. 2018.

[28]   Grimes DA, Schulz KF. Bias and causal associations in observational research. Lancet 2002; 359(9302): 248-52.
[http://dx.doi.org/10.1016/S0140-6736(02)07451-2] [PMID: 11812579]

[29]   Kleinbaum, D. G., Kupper, L. L., & Nizam, A. Epidemiologic Research: Principles and Quantitative Methods. Wiley. 2013.

[30]   Armitage, P., & Berry, G.Statistical Methods in Medical Research. Wiley. 2014.

CHAPTER 4

Disease Surveillance and Outbreak Investigations

Abstract: Chapter 4 offers an extensive exploration of the methodologies and practices involved in monitoring and responding to disease outbreaks. Beginning with an introduction to the themes of the chapter, it delves into the intricacies of disease surveillance systems, providing insights into their establishment and operation. The chapter also examines outbreak detection and response strategies, offering practical guidance on identifying and mitigating emerging health threats. Through compelling case studies, readers gain valuable real-world perspectives on outbreak response efforts, illuminating the challenges and successes encountered in the field of public health.

Keywords: Case Studies, Disease Surveillance, Outbreak Investigations, Outbreak Detection, Response Strategies, Public Health, Surveillance Systems.

INTRODUCTION

In the ever-evolving dance between humanity and infectious diseases, two critical elements play pivotal roles: vigilance and response. The hallmark of modern public health is the ability to detect the emergence of new threats, swiftly identify their patterns, and mount effective interventions. Chapter 4 delves into Disease Surveillance and Outbreak Investigations, where the art and science of tracking diseases and managing epidemics come to life.

Disease surveillance is the silent sentinel of public health, constantly scanning the horizon for signs of trouble. It involves the systematic collection, analysis, interpretation, and dissemination of health data to monitor and understand the dynamics of diseases. Surveillance forms the first line of defence, enabling us to spot anomalies, identify trends, and sound the alarm when danger looms. However, surveillance is not a passive endeavour but an active and dynamic process that demands precision and vigilance.

In this chapter, the journey is into the heart of disease surveillance. It explores the various surveillance systems, from national and global networks to digital tools and crowd-sourced data, that provide us with eyes and ears to detect emerging threats. We will learn about the importance of early warning systems and the role of epidemiologists and public health professionals in curating and interpreting surveillance data.

Nevertheless, the true test of our preparedness comes when the alarm sounds and an outbreak is upon us. Outbreak investigations are the frontlines of the battle against infectious diseases. They are high-stakes endeavours that require swift action, precise methodology, and a collaborative spirit. In this chapter, the discussions will be deep into the art of outbreak investigation, from the initial detection to the formulation of hypotheses and the design of studies that elucidate the source and mode of transmission.

Through case studies and real-world examples, this chapter will examine how outbreak investigations unfold, highlighting the challenges investigators face, the critical role of contact tracing and laboratory diagnostics, and the ethical considerations guiding our response. The reader will also explore the principles of risk communication and crisis management, recognizing that effective communication is as vital as scientific investigation.

In the era of globalization and rapid transportation, infectious diseases can traverse the globe in hours. Disease surveillance and outbreak investigations have become more crucial than ever, demanding innovation and adaptability. The chapter will glimpse into the future of these fields, where genomics, artificial intelligence, and predictive modelling are reshaping our ability to anticipate and control epidemics.

It is critical to remember that disease surveillance and outbreak investigations are not merely academic pursuits; they are the bulwarks that protect our communities and nations from the spectre of pandemics. These tools enable us to respond to crises with agility and compassion, safeguarding lives and preserving the fabric of society. Welcome to a chapter that explores the dynamic world of Disease Surveillance and Outbreak Investigations, where science and action unite to conquer the ever-present threat of infectious diseases.

DISEASE SURVEILLANCE SYSTEMS

Surveillance is critical in epidemiologic practice and is considered an essential feature. The word surveillance, initially limited to infectious diseases but now broadened to cover non-infectious diseases and injuries, was derived from French – **sur**, which means 'over' and **veiller**, which means to 'watch ' [1 - 3]. Surveillance is central in epidemiological practice and helps health officials detect and track diseases, outbreaks of health events, behaviours, and practices that predispose the citizenry to diseases, and biological agents that could be used for bioterrorism. It implies that disease surveillance is a continuous, systematic collection of health data or information about the disease through a systematic approach to be analysed and interpreted. It is the outcome of the analysis, often in the form of reports, that is used to guide in planning, programme implementation, and evaluation of activities [1 - 3].

The surveillance report could be in bulletins or newsletters and can be distributed *via* the following channels - e-mails, postal mail, the webpage of the health department, *etc*. Sharing surveillance reports with the medical community improves collaboration and motivates them to report further. Similarly, the coordinating bodies could share the surveillance reports weekly, monthly, or quarterly (national and subnational levels) for distribution to the local medical and public health communities.

Historical Context

Historically, disease surveillance dates back to the 14th and 15th centuries during the pneumonic plague as a public health measure taken by a government in Europe. During that period, travellers from the plague-infested areas were quarantined for 40 days in Marseilles and Venice to control and prevent the spread of diseases [4 - 6].

In the 16th century, European towns started preserving records of vital events. In 1532, the first London Bills of Mortality were prepared [4, 7].

In the 17th century, the containment strategy of plague in London became one of the earliest examples of surveillance. The parish clerks of London started collecting and sending weekly reports of the number of burials and causes of death to the Hall of the Parish Clerks' Company; this was analysed, interpreted, and disseminated through the weekly "Bill of Mortality" by John Graunt [4, 7, 8].

In the 18th century, Johann Peter Frank pioneered a comprehensive form of public health surveillance in Germany – his attention was on school health, injury prevention, maternal and child health, and public water and sewage treatment [1, 4, 9].

In the 19th century, disease surveillance became fully developed. In England, Sir Edwin Chadwick (1800-90) became the first health administrator to use surveillance and show the relationship between poverty and disease. Similarly, in the U.S., Lemuel Shattuck released a report from the Massachusetts Sanitary Commission" (1850) relating living conditions to infant and maternal mortality and morbidity rates. He recommended a decennial census, standardisation of nomenclature for diseases and causes of death, and collecting health data by age, sex, occupation, socioeconomic level, and locality [4, 7].

In the 20th century, the concept of surveillance and the development of many different surveillance systems were expanded and took centre stage in disease prevention and control [4, 7].

In 1952, the Communicable Disease Center of the US started maintaining a continuous vigilance over serious infectious diseases across the country to enable them to build some level of preparedness to control them adequately them [10].

In 1968, the 21st World Health Assembly defined *surveillance* as "the systematic collection and use of epidemiologic information for the planning, implementation, and assessment of disease control." [11]. Similarly, in the 1980s and 1990s, this definition expanded beyond disease to any outcome, hazard, or exposure [3, 12 - 14].

Definition and Scope

Public health surveillance is defined as the ongoing systematic collection, analysis, and interpretation of health data essential for planning, implementing, and evaluating public health activities [15, 18, 23]. It is critical to note that surveillance covers both communicable and non-communicable diseases; hence, the scope is broad. It supports early warning systems for rapid response in the case of communicable diseases. In contrast, when the health event under surveillance is a chronic disease, it facilitates a planned response because the period between exposure and disease onset is longer.

In line with international requirements, countries have regulations for mandatory reporting of notifiable diseases using their surveillance systems (communicable and non-communicable). These reporting systems have a format that covers both communicable diseases (*e.g.*, vaccine-preventable diseases) and non-communicable diseases (*e.g.*, injuries, maternal deaths, occupational diseases) [15 - 18]. Given that, the uses of surveillance include:

- To detect infectious and non-infectious diseases
- To assess the impact of health events
- To assess trends in health events
- To measure the causal factors of a disease
- To monitor the effectiveness and evaluate the impact of prevention and control measures
- To monitor the effectiveness of intervention strategies and health policy changes
- To use available data to strengthen political commitment and resource mobilization

- To estimate the magnitude of epidemics, monitor trends, and build up an epidemic level of preparedness

It is essential to underscore that surveillance activities are time-bound, hence the need for timely dissemination of information for practical actions. Similarly, the data collected during surveillance activities are evaluated and interpreted to look at disease distribution and trends to help in planning, priority setting, intervention targeting and monitoring, and disease control measures and their effectiveness [19, 20]. The critical surveillance activities to be carried out could be summed up under 5 D:

1. Disease identification: to identify, define, and operationalize how to measure the health event

2. Data collection: to design tools for data collection and compilation

3. Data analysis and interpretation: to analyze and interpret the data for dissemination to relevant authorities

4. Disseminate information: to disseminate the findings to the responsible authorities for controlling the health event

5. Disease monitoring: for continuous monitoring and evaluation to avoid future occurrences.

In surveillance, the data source could be at the national or subnational (state and local) levels. Similarly, gathering surveillance data on the health event of interest could be done through various approaches such as population surveys, notifications on specific diseases, disease registries (population or hospital-based), environmental monitoring, etc [1, 15 - 18].

Types of Surveillance

Having in place an effective surveillance system provides timely, useful evidence that helps decision-makers to lead and manage effectively. Traditionally, there are two types of surveillance: passive and active surveillance. However, in the African region, there is a third type of surveillance referred to as integrated surveillance. The integrated surveillance aims to complement the other two and to serve as an early warning system on the continent for prompt response to emerging and reemerging public health diseases [1, 15 - 18].

1. Passive surveillance: Healthcare providers (clinicians, laboratories, health departments, or other sources) routinely send reports based on set rules and regulations. In this context, there is no active case search. The most used reporting system is routine health management and information systems. The limitations include data completeness and accuracy issues (*e.g.*, whether reporting is legally mandated, the established definitive diagnosis, preference given to more severe illnesses, *etc.*). Some healthcare providers use sentinel reporting. Although the data is of high quality and consistent over time, the sample might not reflect the general population [1, 15 - 18].

2. Active surveillance: Here, the health department initiates the process. In this case, surveillance officers continuously search for cases in the community or health facilities by contacting the reporting source regularly, either physically, to review records or telephone calls. Active surveillance is often limited to specific diseases in a defined population over a limited period (*e.g.*, active search for measles, polio, *etc.*) or during a disease outbreak. Active surveillance can be prospective (through routine contact with reporting sources), retrospective (through audit of hospital records), or combined. The advantage of population-based active surveillance is that it provides the most complete and unbiased disease record because all cases are identified and reported in a given geographic location. However, active surveillance would have limitations, especially when conducted at only one or more participating facilities, as it does not represent the population [1, 15 - 18].

3. Integrated disease surveillance: A standard tool is used to collect health data for multiple disease entities. The aim is to have a robust early warning system for prompt response. The system relies on two main channels of information or signal generation for data collection and analysis: indicator-based surveillance (IBS) and event-based surveillance (EBS) [18].

- *Indicator-based surveillance* uses the following methods:
  - Facility-based surveillance reports weekly, monthly, quarterly, or annually based on the categories of diseases, conditions, and events. In the case of epidemic-prone disease, reporting is immediate.
  - Case-based surveillance is used for diseases targeted for elimination or eradication or during confirmed outbreaks. In this case, any identified case is reported immediately.
  - Sentinel surveillance uses a given number of health facilities or reporting sites to monitor the rate of occurrence of priority events such as pandemic or epidemic events. It represents an area with a risk for a disease or condition of concern (*e.g.*, malaria, meningitis, influenza).
  - Syndromic surveillance uses an active or passive system through a standard case definition based entirely on clinical features (*e.g.*, AFP as an alert for polio, rash, illness as an alert for measles). Here, higher-level reports require

more investigation because of a lack of specificity (see discussion below).

○ Laboratory-based surveillance is conducted at laboratories to detect events or trends. The designated labs can alert for a specific outbreak requiring epidemiological investigations (*e.g.*, antimicrobial resistance).

○ Disease-specific surveillance involves surveillance activities aimed at targeting health data for a specific disease for vertical surveillance (*e.g.*, tuberculosis, malaria, and HIV).

○ Community-based surveillance (CBS) is the systematic detection and reporting of events of public health significance within the community through designated focal persons to the nearest health centres or focal points. It incorporates both indicator-based and event-based surveillance methods using two approaches:

  ▪ Identify and report events based on agreed case definitions (for measles, cholera, polio, and Guinea worm)

  ▪ Reporting of unusual events (alerts) to alert an outbreak or any other public health threat in the community (*e.g.*, unusual animal deaths).

• ***Event-based surveillance*** captures information about events that have potential risks to public health in a timely fashion and is considered part of the early warning and response (EWARS). The alerts, which are triaged and verified before initiating a response, are shared by healthcare workers or community informants and may include:

  ○ Unusual diseases or unexplained deaths

  ○ Health events due to exposure of humans to hazardous substances (*e.g.*, contaminated food products, water, biological, chemical, or radionuclear substances)

  ○ Health events due to natural or man-made disasters.

Addendum: In surveillance, and depending on whether it is general or disease-specific, the data sources include the following:

• Hospital records (out-patient, in-patient, emergency units, physician offices)
• Laboratories,
• Immunization unit (vaccine utilization),
• Medical records department (mortality and morbidity data),
• Blood banks.

Furthermore, to understand the causal chain of the health event or disease of interest (*e.g.*, diseases related to air, water, animal vectors, behavioural actions, *etc.*), the surveillance data could be harvested using the following channels [1, 15 - 17].

1. A **survey** is a method of investigation to obtain specific information using a structured and systematic approach to describe the population of interest quantitatively by sampling a population of interest (*e.g.*, the general public, under-five children, healthcare workers, *etc.*). Surveys are usually conducted once or periodically (*e.g.*, malaria indicator survey, NDHS, *etc.*); the outcome often reflects the general population [21].

2. A **disease notification** is a form of surveillance through reporting specific diseases or a particular health event of interest by disease surveillance and notification officers. These officers are present at the local, state, and national levels. Depending on the level of prioritization, reports are sent daily, weekly, or monthly. However, some diseases are known as notifiable, as required by law for timely control.

3. **Registries** are methods for documenting or tracking events or persons over time (*e.g.*, vital events, cancer, birth, death, *etc.*).

4. **Environmental monitoring** aims to ensure the safety of the environment through qualitative and quantitative approaches (*e.g.*, environmental surveys in polio-endemic countries – Afghanistan, Nigeria, and Pakistan) [22].

However, it is critical to note that human and financial resources often constrain the scope of a surveillance system. Furthermore, this is more so in developing countries, resulting in routine reporting being limited to public health centres and missing out on private and faith-based health centres [10, 16, 17, 23]. This limitation raises questions about the representativeness of the reported surveillance data and whether the surveillance systems could send alerts on outbreaks of national and international concerns. Although developed countries have invested many resources in their surveillance systems, there is a need to support developing countries. This support should ensure the availability of surveillance systems that would timely get data from health facilities at all levels through capacity building and creating and strengthening local capacity to promptly identify and manage effective responses to manage disease outbreaks of national and international concern [17, 24, 25].

Principles and Components

Disease surveillance is a foundational aspect of epidemiology and public health. It involves the systematic collection, analysis, interpretation, and dissemination of health data to monitor and respond to diseases and health events [26]. Effective surveillance systems are built on key principles and consist of various components:

- Principles of Disease Surveillance:
  - Timeliness: Surveillance data should be collected and reported promptly to enable rapid response to emerging health threats.
  - Sensitivity: Surveillance systems should be sensitive enough to detect even small changes in disease occurrence or health events.
  - Specificity: The ability of a system to distinguish between different diseases or health conditions is crucial to avoid misclassification.
  - Flexibility: Surveillance systems must adapt to changing disease patterns and emerging threats.
  - Representativeness: Data should be collected from a representative sample of the population to provide a comprehensive view of health trends.
- Components of Disease Surveillance Systems:
  - Data Collection: Surveillance begins with data collection, which can come from various sources, including healthcare facilities, laboratories, and community reports.
  - Data Analysis: Collected data is analyzed to identify trends, clusters of cases, and potential outbreaks.
  - Data Interpretation: Interpreting data involves determining whether observed trends are significant, and if so, what actions should be taken.
  - Communication: Effective communication of surveillance findings is essential for informing public health actions and policymaking.
  - Response: When surveillance identifies a health threat or outbreak, public health agencies must respond promptly to contain and mitigate the impact.

Real-Time Monitoring

Advancements in technology have enabled real-time monitoring and reporting of health data. This approach allows for the continuous and immediate collection and analysis of health information. Real-time monitoring systems are particularly valuable in responding to rapidly spreading diseases and emerging health threats [27].

Exercise 1: Analyzing Local Disease Surveillance Data

In this exercise, readers will gain hands-on experience in analyzing local disease surveillance data:

- Access Local Disease Surveillance Data: Obtain access to disease surveillance data specific to your region or community. This data may include information on disease incidence, prevalence, or outbreak reports.

- Select a Health Issue: Choose a specific health issue or disease of interest from the available surveillance data. It could be a recent outbreak or a long-term health trend.
- Analyze the Data: Use appropriate statistical and epidemiological methods to analyze the data. Calculate key measures such as incidence rate, prevalence, and trends over time.
- Interpret the Findings: Interpret the results of your analysis. Are there any notable trends or patterns in the data? Are there areas of concern or areas where public health efforts have been successful?
- Prepare a Report: Create a concise report summarizing your findings. Include relevant statistics, charts, and tables. Discuss the implications of your analysis for public health practice or policy.
- Present Your Findings: Present your report to a group or class to practice effectively communicating surveillance findings.

This exercise empowers readers to engage with real-world disease surveillance data, apply epidemiological principles, and make informed assessments of local health issues. It reinforces the practical application of disease surveillance in public health practice.

SETTING UP A SURVEILLANCE SYSTEM

Epidemiologists have underscored the importance of an effective surveillance system that can directly measure what is happening in the population. It is important to note that public health problems vary based on geographical settings. Thus, a malaria outbreak in the US or Europe could be a public health emergency, while Africa is considered a stable transmission. Similarly, while some diseases could pose a threat and require immediate attention (*e.g.*, polio, influenza epidemics, COVID-19 pandemic), others could have a relatively stable incidence and prevalence (*e.g.*, hypertension, diabetes, breast cancer) [1, 15 - 17].

For a surveillance system to be valuable and cost-effective, it is necessary to develop a clear description and diagram of surveillance activities, identify and include key stakeholders in the evaluation processes, and assess the usefulness, resource requirements, and characteristics of optimal surveillance. Therefore, an ideal surveillance system should be clear on the following [1, 15].

- Case definition
- Purpose and objectives
- Planned uses of the collected data
- Ethical/legal concerns
- Stand-alone or integrated with other surveillance systems

- Population
- Frequency of data collection (daily, weekly, monthly, annually)
- Source of data
- Approach to data collection (passive, active)
- Data management (confidentiality, processing, analysis)
- Dissemination of findings (bulletins, advocacy, policymakers, medical and public health communities).

Likewise, the key attributes of a robust surveillance system include [1,16]:

- Quality of the data (to reflect completeness and validity)
- Sensitive to pick up cases
- Specific in picking up non-cases
- Representativeness of the true population (findings should portray the disease incidence among the population)
- Timeliness in data collection and providing feedback (to the data providers, community, and policymakers)
- Validity to measure what it is intended to measure to rightly detect an outbreak (related to sensitivity and positive predictive value)
- Positive predictive value (to ensure that a proportion of the cases are true cases, or it is truly an epidemic/pandemic to avoid false positives, wasting resources)
- Stability (reliability of computer systems and availability of human and capital resources)
- Acceptability through the willingness of persons and organizations to participate in the surveillance activities (time, effort to complete and submit reports)
- Flexibility to make provision to accommodate changes without distorting the system (tools, personnel, funds)

Using a standard case definition for surveillance is critical in epidemiological practice. A case definition uses a set of standard criteria to classify whether an individual has a particular disease in question [15, 17, 23]. However, in the context of case definition and while waiting for the laboratory results to become available, a case could be classified as suspected, probable, or confirmed. In an ideal setting, it is laboratory investigations that would establish the status of a case. However, a standard case definition must be universally acceptable and ensure that every case is equivalent, irrespective of race, gender, or geographical location. However, when dealing with a disease outbreak situation, the case definition could be tailored within the local context; this ranges from simple clinical signs and symptoms (*e.g.*, bacterial pneumonia in children in a resource-lacking setting could be based only on a physical examination using the WHO guidelines) to as complex conducting some laboratory confirmation (*e.g.*, the case definition for AIDS should in HIV-infected individuals require a CD4+ T-lymphocyte count of less than 200 per microlitre) where applicable [15, 21]. Similarly, diagnostic criteria change with additional information about a disease or the availability of diagnostic techniques (*e.g.*, initial WHO diagnostic criteria for myocardial infarction were modified in 1980 with the introduction of an objective method for assessing electrocardiograms; this also changed in the 1990s, when measuring cardiac enzymes became available) [20, 28, 29].

Evaluating the surveillance system should be a periodic process, and the goal is to assess the system's sensitivity. The evaluation process helps alert the public health alert warning system to meet its objectives. The evaluation process of the surveillance system aims to identify the critical elements and data quality to give insight into the system's effectiveness [1]. simple way to evaluate the surveillance system is by identifying and interviewing key stakeholders, collecting background documents (forms and reports), the mechanics of conducting surveillance, and the resources needed. The outcome is expected to provide recommendations for improvement where needed [1].

OUTBREAK DETECTION AND RESPONSE

Identifying Outbreaks

Outbreak detection is a critical function of disease surveillance systems. It involves recognizing unusual or unexpected patterns of illness that may indicate the occurrence of an outbreak. Key steps in identifying outbreaks include [30].

- Surveillance Data Analysis: Continuously monitor surveillance data for spikes or clusters of cases that exceed expected levels.
- Thresholds and Alarms: Establish threshold levels for specific diseases or health events. When data surpasses these thresholds, it triggers an alarm for further investigation.
- Epidemiological Clues: Look for epidemiological clues such as common exposures or risk factors among cases.
- Laboratory Confirmation: Laboratory tests may confirm the presence of a specific pathogen, further supporting outbreak suspicion.

Epidemiologists interchangeably use the words outbreak and epidemic to refer to the occurrence of more cases than expected in each population over some time. In simpler terms, an *outbreak* could be defined as an epidemic limited to a localised increase in the incidence of a disease in a smaller community, *e.g.*, a village, town, or institution. However, to the broader audience, an epidemic points to a crisis. Health departments uncover outbreaks through routine review of surveillance data; this is done regularly, timely analysis of surveillance data for an increase in reported cases, and observing unusual health events by clinicians, infection control practitioners, or laboratories in isolation or clusters. In some instances, patients or community members may call the health, informing them that there is an unusual health event (*e.g.*, diarrhoea after attending a night party with a friend) or women giving birth to babies with defects in a particular community [1, 15 - 17]. In a simpler form, the ABCs for determining a disease outbreak are:

- *Alert the system* about higher than usual number of a specific disease (*e.g.*, shigellosis from weekly reports, pneumonia from nursing homes)
- *Be clear* about the normal estimate for "usual" or "unusual."
- *Confirm* if the health event is higher than usual
- *Describe* whether the reported cases should be called suspected "cluster," "an outbreak," or "an epidemic?"
- *Ensure* to agree on criteria for field investigations and how to conduct the investigation.

Investigation Protocols

When an outbreak is suspected, public health authorities initiate a structured investigation process to identify the source, implement control measures, and prevent further spread. The main goal of outbreak investigation is to learn about the disease situation and promptly implement appropriate control and prevention measures. Depending on the situation, other reasons include learning more about the disease, the causative agent, the associated risk factors, safeguarding public lives, and legal and political concerns. Similarly, it serves as an avenue to evaluate the health systems' effectiveness and level of preparedness [1, 15 - 17, 31, 32].

When dealing with a suspected disease outbreak, the decisions to investigate often depend on a variety of factors:

- Health problems (*e.g.*, severity, cases, mode of transmission, the existence of control measures)
- Health department (*e.g.*, availability of staff, resources, other competing priorities)
- External concerns (*e.g.*, potential to spread further in the absence of prompt control measures)

Nonetheless, the need to conduct outbreak investigations must be considered as it allows epidemiologists to conduct research, train public health personnel, and, most importantly, for public health considerations. The lead epidemiologist should adopt a *systematic approach* for the *positive predictive outcome*. The team should use the local data for guidance and get the background information of the area (if absent, conduct a community survey to establish the background or historical level of the disease) [1, 15 - 17].

The following steps for *Outbreak Investigations* are considered conceptual and give room for the investigators to decide on a different approach that suits them:

- Planning meetings with stakeholders (MoH, national CDC, WHO, UNICEF, *etc.*)
- Constitute Emergency Operation Centre: *e.g.*, Incident Manager, Administrative, Managerial, Logistics, Communication Specialist, *etc.*
- Constitute Outbreak Investigation Team: *e.g.*, Epidemiologist, DSNO, Laboratorian, Veterinarian, Translator/Interpreter, Computer Specialist, Entomologist, Local Officers, *etc.*)
- Identify requirements for the fieldwork (*e.g.*, scientific literature on suspected disease, administrative staff, investigation tools, guidance on sample collection, storage and transportation techniques, logistics, and equipment such as PPEs)
- Confirm the outbreak (is it a cluster of cases, an outbreak, or an epidemic? The numerator will guide you in this regard)
- Confirm the diagnosis (clinical and laboratory approach)
- Develop a workable case definition.
- Create a database: line list cases, organize the data by time, place, and person, and update the record systematically.
- Use a Descriptive Epidemiological approach to look at the disease distribution (to help characterize the outbreak, identify the population at risk, develop hypotheses about risk factors, to help target control and prevention strategies)
- Develop hypotheses (using the disease information and what others postulated)
- Conduct Analytic study (in some outbreaks, using either a cohort (comparing attack rates with risk ratios to identify associations) or a case-control (compute an odds ratio to look for associations) studies to identify associations between exposures (risk factors or causes) and the disease of interest.
- Implement control and prevention measures (NB: often done in the early stage; establish the link in the transmission chain, the source and mode of transmission)
- Communicate the findings effectively.
- Maintain the surveillance system in place (to ensure the effectiveness of the control measures and avoid resurgence).

Though critical when conducting outbreak investigations, these steps listed may only sometimes be applied. It is important to note that the hallmark of outbreak investigations is to institute effective control and preventive measures and to disseminate the findings effectively. The report, which gives details on the outcome of the disease outbreak, should be shared with the relevant stakeholders in a timely and regular fashion. The stakeholders include the community, partners, providers of the data (health facilities, laboratories), and policymakers (for health-related decision-making and prevention and control strategies) [1, 15 - 17].

Thus, in summary, the investigation protocol typically includes [33]:

- Case Definition: Define and standardize what constitutes a confirmed case of the disease under investigation.
- Case Finding: Identify and confirm cases using surveillance data, healthcare records, laboratory results, and clinical assessments.
- Hypothesis Generation: Develop initial hypotheses about the source of the outbreak, potential exposures, and modes of transmission.
- Epidemiological Studies: Conduct epidemiological studies, such as case-control or cohort studies, to test hypotheses and identify commonalities among cases.
- Environmental Assessment: Investigate potential environmental sources, such as contaminated food or water, to pinpoint the outbreak's origin.
- Control Measures: Implement control measures to contain the outbreak, which may include isolation, quarantine, treatment, or vaccination.
- Communication: Communicate findings to the public, healthcare providers, and relevant authorities to raise awareness and facilitate coordinated responses.

Exercise 2: Conducting Outbreak Investigations in Your Region

In this exercise, readers will practice conducting outbreak investigations in their region or community:

- Select a Local Outbreak: Choose a recent or historical outbreak that occurred in your region. It could be related to a foodborne illness, infectious disease, or any other health event.
- Define Your Investigation Objectives: Clearly define the objectives of your investigation. What specific questions do you want to answer? What are your goals in investigating this outbreak?
- Gather Relevant Data: Collect data related to the outbreak, including case reports, medical records, laboratory results, and exposure histories.
- Develop a Case Definition: Create a case definition for the outbreak to standardize case identification.

- Analyze the Data: Apply epidemiological methods to analyze the data, such as calculating attack rates, identifying risk factors, and generating hypotheses.
- Conduct Interviews: If possible, conduct interviews with affected individuals to gather additional information on exposures and symptoms.
- Formulate Hypotheses: Develop hypotheses about the outbreak's source, mode of transmission, and contributing factors.
- Report and Communicate: Prepare a report summarizing your findings and recommendations for control measures. Practice effective communication of outbreak investigation results.

This exercise provides a hands-on opportunity for readers to apply outbreak investigation principles to a local or regional context. It reinforces the importance of rapid response, collaboration, and evidence-based decision-making in outbreak management.

CASE STUDIES IN OUTBREAK RESPONSE

Notable Outbreaks and Lessons Learned

The field of epidemiology is replete with examples of outbreaks that have shaped public health practices and policies. Case studies of notable outbreaks offer valuable insights into the challenges faced, innovations in response, and lessons learned. Some well-known outbreaks include [34].

1. Ebola Outbreak (2014-2016): This West African epidemic highlighted the need for international cooperation and rapid response to contain highly infectious diseases.

2. SARS Outbreak (2002-2003): Severe Acute Respiratory Syndrome demonstrated the potential for global spread and the importance of early detection and containment.

3. HIV/AIDS Pandemic: The ongoing HIV/AIDS pandemic has underscored the importance of long-term surveillance, prevention strategies, and access to treatment.

4. E. coli O157:H7 Outbreak (1993): The Jack in the Box outbreak in the U.S. led to improved food safety regulations and practices.

Challenges and Innovations

Each outbreak presents unique challenges, but common themes emerge, including the need for rapid response, effective communication, and coordination among healthcare professionals and agencies. Innovations in outbreak response include [35].

1. Genomic Epidemiology: The use of genomics to track the evolution of pathogens and identify sources of infection.

2. Vaccination Campaigns: Mass vaccination campaigns to control diseases like polio and measles.

3. Digital Surveillance: Utilizing digital tools and data sources for real-time monitoring and early detection.

4. Antimicrobial Stewardship: Strategies to combat antibiotic resistance by promoting responsible antibiotic use.

Exercise 3: Developing Outbreak Response Plans for Local Challenges

In this exercise, readers will develop outbreak response plans tailored to local challenges.

- Identify Local Health Challenges: Research and identify specific health challenges or potential outbreak scenarios in your region or community. Consider local demographics, environmental factors, and healthcare infrastructure.
- Review Case Studies: Study one or more case studies of past outbreaks, preferably those that share similarities with the identified local challenges. Analyze the strategies and lessons from these outbreaks.
- Develop Response Plans: Based on the lessons learned from the case studies, we create outbreak response plans for the identified local challenges. Outline key steps, roles and responsibilities, communication strategies, and resource requirements.
- Scenario Testing: Simulate outbreak scenarios and test the effectiveness of your response plan. Consider the different variables and challenges that may arise during an outbreak.
- Feedback and Refinement: Seek feedback from peers or experts in epidemiology and public health. Refine your response plan based on feedback and additional research.
- Presentation: Present your outbreak response plan to a group or class to practice communicating and defending your strategies.

This exercise empowers readers to apply knowledge gained from case studies to real-world outbreak response planning. It emphasizes the importance of adaptability and preparedness in the face of evolving health challenges.

CONCLUSION

In conclusion, Chapter 4 has offered a comprehensive exploration of disease surveillance and outbreak investigations, highlighting the methodologies and practices essential for monitoring and responding to health threats. By examining disease surveillance systems, outbreak detection strategies, and real-world case studies, readers have gained valuable insights into the dynamic nature of public health surveillance and response efforts. Moreover, the chapter underscores the importance of proactive surveillance measures and coordinated response strategies in mitigating the impact of disease outbreaks. As readers continue through subsequent chapters, they will further deepen their understanding of disease surveillance and outbreak management, contributing to the advancement of public health practice and policy.

REFERENCES

[1]   An Introduction to Applied Epidemiology and Biostatistics. Principles of Epidemiology in Public Health Practice. 3rd ed. Atlanta, GA: Centres for Disease Control and Prevention 2012; p. 30333.

[2]   Langmuir AD. The surveillance of communicable diseases of national importance. N Engl J Med 1963; 268(4): 182-92.
[http://dx.doi.org/10.1056/NEJM196301242680405] [PMID: 13928666]

[3]   Thacker SB, Berkelman RL. Public health surveillance in the United States. Epidemiol Rev 1988; 10(1): 164-90.
[http://dx.doi.org/10.1093/oxfordjournals.epirev.a036021] [PMID: 3066626]

[4]   Declich S, Carter AO. Public health surveillance: historical origins, methods and evaluation. Bull World Health Organ 1994; 72(2): 285-304.
[PMID: 8205649]

[5]   Evans AS. Surveillance and seroepidemiology. In: Evans AS, Ed. Viral infections of humans. New York: Plenum Press 1982; pp. 43-64.
[http://dx.doi.org/10.1007/978-1-4613-3237-4_2]

[6]   Moro ML, McCormick A. Surveillance for communicable disease. In: Eylenbosh WJ, Noah ND, Eds. Surveillance in health and disease. Oxford: Oxford University Press 1988; pp. 166-82.

[7]   Eylenbosch WJ, Noah ND, Eds. Surveillance in health and disease. Oxford: Oxford University Press 1988.

[8]   Galbraith NS. Communicable disease surveillance. In: Smith A, Ed. Recent advances in community medicine, No 2. London: Churchill Livingstone 1982; pp. 127-42.

[9]   Editorials. Int J Epidemiol 1976; 5(1): 3-7.
[http://dx.doi.org/10.1093/ije/5.1.3] [PMID: 1262109]

[10]   1953.

[11]   Report of the technical discussions at the twenty-first World Health Assembly on 'national and global surveillance of communicable diseases. Geneva: World Health Organization 1968.

[12]   Thacker SB, Stroup DF, Parrish RG, Anderson HA. Surveillance in environmental public health: issues, systems, and sources. Am J Public Health 1996; 86(5): 633-8.
[http://dx.doi.org/10.2105/AJPH.86.5.633] [PMID: 8629712]

[13]   Vaughan JP, Morrow RH. Manual of epidemiology for district health management. Geneva: World Health Organization 1989.

[14] Wegman DH. Hazard Surveillance. In: Halperin W, Baker E, Monson R, Eds. Public Health Surveillance. New York: Van Nostrand Reinhold 1992.

[15] Bonita R, Beaglehole R, Kjellström T. Basic epidemiology. 2nd ed., World Health Organ 2006.

[16] McNamara LA, Martin SW. Principles of Epidemiology and Public Health. Principles and Practice of Pediatric Infectious Diseases. 5th ed. Philadelphia, PA: Elsevier 2018; pp. 19103-2899.
[http://dx.doi.org/10.1016/B978-0-323-40181-4.00001-3]

[17] Clements BW. Bioterrorism. Disasters and Public Health. Butterworth-Heinemann 2009; pp. 27-63.
[http://dx.doi.org/10.1016/B978-1-85617-612-5.00007-X]

[18] Technical Guidelines for Integrated Disease Surveillance and Response in the African Region. 3rd ed., Brazzaville: WHO Regional Office for Africa 2019.

[19] 1995.The management of acute respiratory infections in children.

[20] Recomm Rep MMWR. Revised Classification System for HIV Infection and Expanded Surveillance Case Definition for AIDS Among Adolescents and Adults 1993; 1992: 41.

[21] Saleh JEA, Saddiq A, Uchenna AA. LLIN Ownership, Utilization, and Malaria Prevalence: An Outlook at the 2015 Nigeria Malaria Indicator Survey. OAlib 2018; 5(1): 1-12.
[http://dx.doi.org/10.4236/oalib.1104280]

[22] Guidelines for environmental surveillance of poliovirus circulation www.who.int/vaccines-documents/

[23] Githinji S, Oyando R, Malinga J, *et al.* Completeness of malaria indicator data reporting *via* the District Health Information Software 2 in Kenya, 2011–2015. Malar J 2017; 16(1): 344.
[http://dx.doi.org/10.1186/s12936-017-1973-y] [PMID: 28818071]

[24] Kiberu VM, Matovu JKB, Makumbi F, Kyozira C, Mukooyo E, Wanyenze RK. Strengthening district-based health reporting through the district health management information software system: the Ugandan experience. BMC Med Inform Decis Mak 2014; 14(1): 40.
[http://dx.doi.org/10.1186/1472-6947-14-40] [PMID: 24886567]

[25] Maïga A, Jiwani SS, Mutua MK, *et al.* Generating statistics from health facility data: the state of routine health information systems in Eastern and Southern Africa. BMJ Global Health Journal 2019; 4: p. e001849.
[http://dx.doi.org/10.1136/bmjgh-2019-001849]

[26] Gregg MB, Ed. Field Epidemiology. 3rd ed., Oxford University Press 2008.
[http://dx.doi.org/10.1093/acprof:oso/9780195313802.001.0001]

[27] Henning KJ. What is syndromic surveillance? MMWR Suppl 2004; 53 (Suppl.): 5-11.
[PMID: 15714620]

[28] Luepker RV, Evans A, McKeigue P, Reddy KS. Cardiovascular Survey Methods. 3rd ed., Geneva: World Health Organization 2004.

[29] Antman E, Bassand J-P, Klein W, *et al.* Myocardial infarction redefined—a consensus document of The Joint European Society of Cardiology/American College of Cardiology committee for the redefinition of myocardial infarction. J Am Coll Cardiol 2000; 36(3): 959-69.
[http://dx.doi.org/10.1016/S0735-1097(00)00804-4] [PMID: 10987628]

[30] Principles of Epidemiology in Public Health Practice. 3rd ed., U.S. Department of Health & Human Services 2012.

[31] Saleh JEA, Wondimagegnehu A, Mpazanje R, Ozor L, Abdullahi S. Investigation of a Suspected Malaria Outbreak in Sokoto State, Nigeria, 2016. OAlib 2017; 4(12): 1-8.
[http://dx.doi.org/10.4236/oalib.1104246]

[32] Saleh JEA, Saddiq A, Adamu HI, Mpazanje R, Audu BM. Suspected Malaria Outbreak Investigations in Baure LGA, Katsina State, Nigeria. OAlib 2019; 6(7): 1-7.
[http://dx.doi.org/10.4236/oalib.1105512]

[33]   Field Guide: Outbreak Investigation, Response and Evaluation in the African Region. WHO Regional Office for Africa 2008.

[34]   Heymann DL, Ed. Control of Communicable Diseases Manual. 20th ed., American Public Health Association 2014.

[35]   Swerdlow DL, Finelli L. Preparation for possible avian influenza pandemic. Emerg Infect Dis 2006; 12(2): 159-63.

CHAPTER 5

Statistical Methods

Abstract: Chapter 5 provides an in-depth exploration of the foundational concepts and tools essential for statistical analysis in epidemiology. Beginning with an introduction to the themes of the chapter, it delves into fundamental statistical measures and inference techniques, equipping readers with the skills needed to interpret and analyze epidemiological data. Moreover, the chapter examines mathematical modelling approaches used to forecast disease trends and inform public health interventions. Through a comprehensive examination of these statistical methods, readers gain a deeper understanding of their applications in epidemiological research and practice.

Keywords: Analysis Techniques, Epidemiological Data, Mathematical Modeling, Public Health, Statistical Methods, Statistical Measures, Statistical Inference.

INTRODUCTION

In our journey through the captivating landscape of epidemiology, we have traced the origins, studied the models, explored research design, and dived into the realm of disease surveillance and outbreak investigations. Now, as we ascend the intellectual summit of this scientific discipline, we arrive at a critical juncture—Chapter 5, where the art of data analysis takes centre stage. Welcome to the world of Statistical Methods.

Statistical methods are the alchemy of epidemiology, transformative processes that turn raw data into knowledge, uncertainty into understanding, and chaos into clarity. In this chapter, we embark on a voyage through mathematical and analytical tools that empower epidemiologists to draw meaningful conclusions from the complex tapestry of disease data.

We begin by unravelling the fundamental concepts of statistics, demystifying terms like probability, hypothesis testing, and confidence intervals. These are not mere mathematical abstractions but the linguistic currency of scientific inquiry. As we delve deeper, the reader will discover the power of these statistical concepts in illuminating the hidden patterns of disease transmission, uncovering risk factors, and evaluating the effectiveness of public health interventions.

In epidemiology, data come in many forms—surveys, case reports, laboratory results, and more. Statistical methods provide tools to wrangle this diverse data into submission, transforming it into actionable insights [1 - 3]. We will explore the art of data management, data visualization, and exploratory data analysis, enabling us to understand the characteristics and peculiarities of our datasets. However, statistical methods are not just about organizing and visualizing data; they are the engines that drive our inferential machinery. We will journey through statistical tests, from the humble t-test to formidable regression models, witnessing how these methods allow us to draw inferences about populations based on samples and quantify the strength of associations between variables [1 - 3].

In the age of big data, where terabytes of information flow in real-time from digital sources and sensors, statistical methods are undergoing a renaissance. We will have a glimpse of the future of epidemiology, where machine learning algorithms, Bayesian modelling, and data-driven decision-making are reshaping our ability to predict disease outbreaks, tailor interventions, and allocate resources efficiently [1 - 3]. As we venture into this chapter, remember that statistics is not a dry mathematical exercise—it is the language of evidence in epidemiology. The integrity of our findings, the validity of our conclusions, and the impact of our research hinge on the sound application of statistical methods. In an era where data are often referred to as the new oil, statistical proficiency is the refinery that turns data into insights.

Welcome to Chapter 5, where we navigate the intricate world of Statistical Methods, unlocking the power to extract knowledge from data, discern signals from noise, and provide the empirical foundation upon which public health decisions are made. This is where the art and science of epidemiology culminate, where data and analysis unite to illuminate the path toward a healthier future [1 - 5].

In the epidemiological context, epidemiologists need to understand a variable, how to effectively handle and process data, how to master the art of tabulating data, how to create databases, and how to plot graphs.

A ***variable*** is any characteristic that differentiates one person from another (*e.g.,* sex, height, vaccination status, employed, or unemployed).

Similarly, a variable may have the value of a number or descriptor (male, married, vaccinated), and this influences the way it is summarized. Therefore, variables, depending on their scale of measurements, can broadly be classified into *Categorical and Numerical*. The categorical class has *nominal* and *ordinal,* while the numerical class has a *ratio* and *interval* [1, 5 - 8].

Categorical

Nominal scale, considered qualitative or categorical, has values in categories without any numerical ranking (*e.g.*, married/single/divorced or alive/dead). A dichotomous variable is a nominal variable with two mutually exclusive categories (yes or no, dead or alive, ill or well).

Ordinal scale, also considered qualitative or categorical, has ranked values (*e.g.*, 1,2,3, or is classified into categories, such as blood groups A, B, O, AB).

Numerical

Interval scale, considered quantitative or continuous, has values that are measured on an equally spaced interval and without a true zero point (*e.g.*, weight, height, age range of children such as 0-5, 6-10, 11-15, *etc.*).

Ratio scale, also considered quantitative or continuous, has values within an interval and with a true zero point (*e.g.*, 1.60, 1.80, 2.20).

CONCEPTS AND TOOLS

Epidemiologists must have a sound knowledge of basic biostatistics and understand the concepts and tools. It is a prerequisite that epidemiologists understand the basic steps and ways of summarizing and analyzing data. Equally important is mastering ways to interpret and communicate the findings effectively. The basic ways include using simple tables (rows and columns) and graphs (showing trends and distributions). While tables and graphs are essential for descriptive and analytical epidemiology, selecting the right samples and confidence intervals are considered critical estimation tools for testing hypotheses. There are various ways of summarizing data [1 - 3, 5]:

1. A **Table**, considering the foundation for generating graphs and charts, presents data in rows and columns. Descriptive epidemiology is considered a basic step in organizing quantitative information; hence, there is a need to make it as simple as possible, as shown in Table **1** [1 - 3, 5]. The data in the table are organized using an epidemiologic database with titles, rows, and columns. In the rows are records or observations representing a person or a case, and in the columns are variables representing characteristics of the person, such as race, gender, and date of birth.

The data are captured in a table such that the first column is for name or ID, followed by demographic information, clinical details, source of exposure, diagnosis, *etc*. Depending on the number of variables, three basic types of tables are used in descriptive epidemiology – one, two, and three-variable tables. Examples of these tables are shown below. A **one-variable table** presents information about one variable, *e.g.*, 'age group', showing the number of food poisonings in a report, as shown in Table **2a**.

Table 1. The frequency distribution of reported measles in a rural village (2015-19).

Year	Reported Measles Cases	-
2015	15	-
2016	12	-
2017	32	-
2018	13	-
2019	9	-

Table 2a. Reported food poisoning in a high school in a state in country X in 2015.

Age Group (yrs)	Reported Cases
<14	3
15–19	12
20–24	23
≥25	4
Total	42

However, the table can also be modified to show percentages and or cumulative percentages in separate columns, as shown in Tables **2b** and **2c**.

Table 2b. Reported food poisoning in a high school in a state in country X in 2015.

Age Group (yrs)	Reported Cases	Percent
<14	3	7.14
15–19	12	28.57
20–24	23	54.76
≥25	4	9.52
Total	42	100.00

Table 2c. Reported food poisoning in a high school in a state in country X in 2015.

Age Group (yrs)	Reported Cases	Percent	Cumulative Percent
<14	3	7.14	7.14
15–19	12	28.57	35.71
20–24	23	54.76	90.48
≥25	4	9.52	100.00

(Table 2c) cont.....

Age Group (yrs)	Reported Cases	Percent	Cumulative Percent
Total	42	100.00	100.00

A **two-variable table** presents information about two variables, *e.g.*, 'age group' and 'sex' in a food poisoning report, as shown in Table **3**.

Table 3. Reported food poisoning in a high school in a state in country X in 2015.

Age Group (yrs)	Reported Cases		-
	Male	Female	Total
<14	2	1	3
15–19	7	5	12
20–24	11	12	23
≥25	2	2	4
Total	22	20	42

2. Graph/chart displays numeric data visually in patterns, distribution, or trends. It is also considered an essential tool to analyze and make sense of data. Designing graphs has the same approach with tables – title, identify variables, legend or keys, and units. It is advisable to assign the dependent variable (frequency) on the y-axis and the independent variable (time or age) on the x-axis, labelling axis. Some of the most famous graphs used in epidemiological studies include bar charts, pie charts, histograms, line graphs, etc, whose examples are given below [1,2,3,5]:

i. **Bar chart** displays comparative data using bars of equal width as in Fig (**1**). There is also a grouped bar chart that illustrates data from two or three-variable tables, as shown in Figs. (**2** and **3**)

ii. **Pie chart** uses slices or wedges to show the contribution of each component part in a proportional manner, as shown in Figs. (**4a** and **b**).

iii. **Histogram** is a graphical presentation of a frequency distribution of a continuous variable using class intervals, as shown in Fig. (**5**).

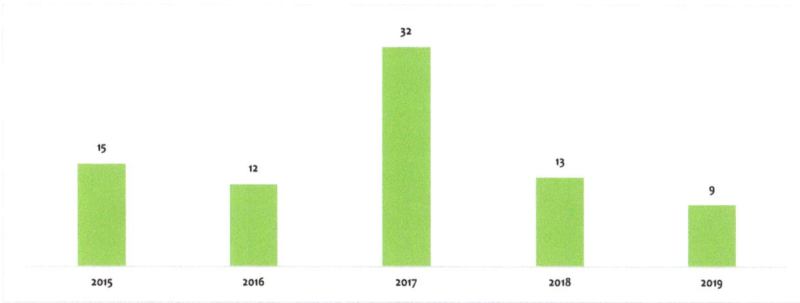

Fig. (1). An example of a simple bar chart of reported measles in a rural village in country X (2015-19).

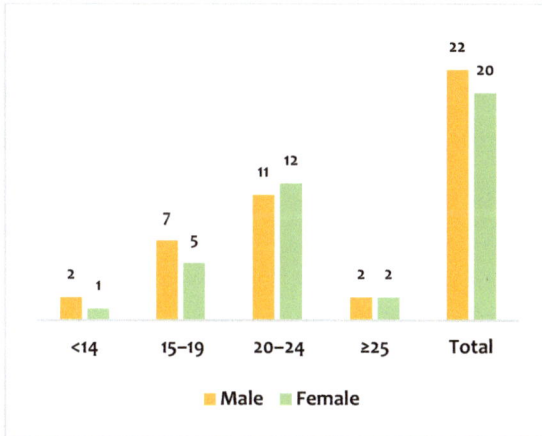

Fig. (2). An example of a bar chart using data from Table **3**.

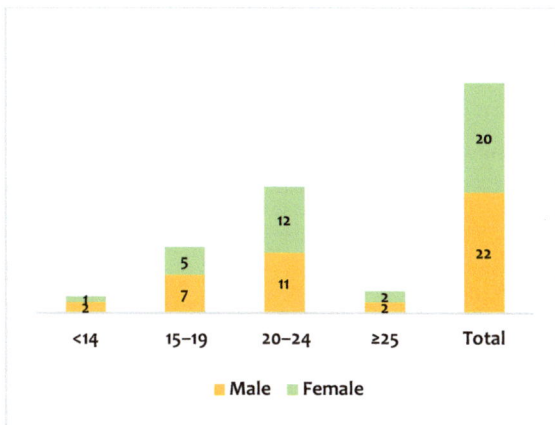

Fig. (3). An example of a stacked bar chart using data from Table **3**.

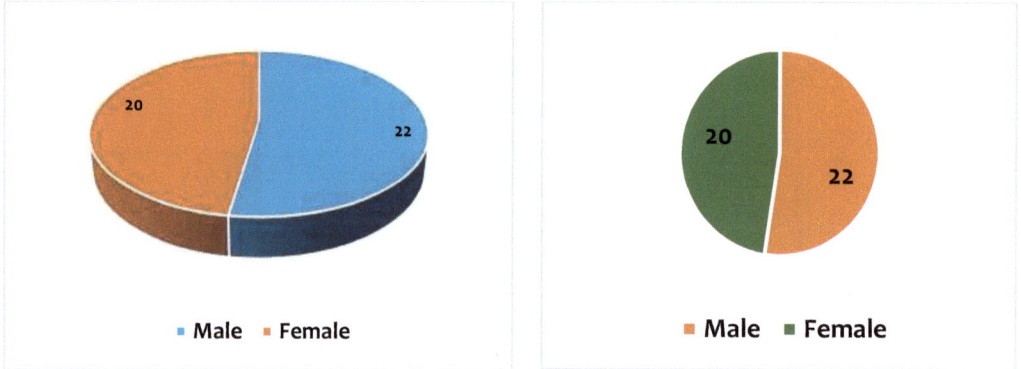

Fig. (4a & b). An example of a pie chart in two dimensions (3D and 2D) using information from Table **3**.

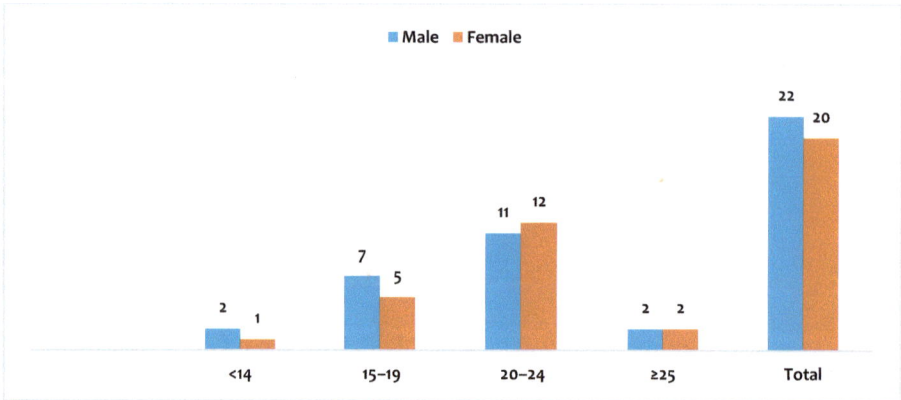

Fig. (5). An example of a histogram using information from Table **3**.

Another example of a two-variable table is shown in Table **4**.

Table 4. COVID-19 cases in country X reported in 2020.

Age Group (yrs)	Reported Cases	
	Male	Female
0-4	88	-63
5-9	113	-98
10-14	132	-101
15-19	197	-123
20-24	203	-147
25-29	254	-178
30-34	334	-204
35-39	357	-237

(Table 4) cont.....

Age Group (yrs)	Reported Cases	
	Male	Female
40-44	344	-244
45-49	376	-289
50-54	398	-302
55-59	401	-301
60-64	202	-126
65-69	102	-42
70-74	69	-32
>75	92	-67

Similarly, when the data are jointly categorized by two variables in a Two-Variable Table, it is referred to as a **contingency table,** as shown in Table **5.**

Table 5. Examples of a Two-by-Two Contingency Table.

Ill	Not Ill	Total
A (40)	B (8)	A+B (48)
C (10)	D (35)	C+D (45)
A+C (50)	B+D (43)	93

A **three-variable table** presents information about three variables, *e.g.*, 'age group' and 'sex' in a food poisoning report as in Table **6**. However, understanding a three-variable table is not as easy as the one- and two-variable tables.

Table 6. Reported food poisoning in a high school in a state in country X in 2015.

Location of residence	Age Group (yrs)	Reported Cases		-
		Male	Female	Total
District A	<14	1	1	2
	15–19	2	3	5
	20–24	5	7	12
	≥25	0	1	1
	Total	8	12	20
District B	<14	0	0	0
	15–19	1	1	2
	20–24	3	2	5
	≥25	0	0	0

(Table 6) cont.....

| Location of residence | Age Group (yrs) | Reported Cases | | - |
		Male	Female	Total
	Total	4	3	7
District C	<14	1	0	1
	15–19	4	1	5
	20–24	3	3	6
	≥25	2	1	3
	Total	10	5	15

i. **Line graph** displays information by a segmented straight line connecting the data points. A line graph is often used to display trends over time, *e.g.*, in time series, as shown in Fig. (**6**).

i. **Other graphical displays** that are critical for the epidemiologist to know how to construct and interpret them include:

   a. A **scatter plot** is a mathematical diagram that uses Cartesian coordinates to display values for two continuous variables of a given data set. It describes the relationship between two continuous variables, and the interpretations are - positive correlation, negative or inverse correlation, and little correlation. The statistical tool used is linear regression and displays correlation to answer causal relationships as in Fig. (**7**) [1 - 4, 9].

   b. **Dot (and box) plots** use data points to show the relationship between a categorical and a continuous variable on the x and y-axis. They are used for continuous, quantitative data, plotted on a simple scale, and summarized using "box and whiskers" as in Fig. (**8**) [1 - 4, 10].

   c. **Phylogenetic tree**, also known as an evolutionary tree, shows the evolutionary relationships of microorganisms (phylogeny), especially during outbreaks. The distance between the nodes infers genetic differences. The relationships are interpreted by looking at the distance between the nodes on the tree – closer ones are more related than the furthest ones [1 - 4].

   d. **Decision tree** is an analytical tool using branches to represent a logical sequence or pathway to public health or clinical decision-making, as shown in Fig. (**9**). Often used in operational research, decision analysis, and when the outcomes are not certain, the building blocks are - decisions (on the type of action to take), outcomes (follows a decision), resource costs, and probabilities. The building blocks are used to represent and examine complex decision problems using an algorithm that contains conditional control statements. The sum of probabilities for the outcomes to occur at a chance node is one [1 - 4, 11, 12].

e. **Maps** are another way of displaying the geographical location of events. Maps could be presented either as spot maps or area maps, as shown in Fig. (**10**). While a spot map shows the geographic distribution of cases, it is short of giving information on the size of the population at risk. However, an area map shows rates of a disease or health event of interest in different areas using colours or shades [1 - 4].

f. **Population pyramid**, also called a pyramid chart, is typically used when dealing with data about a group of individuals based on age and sex, as in Fig. (**11**). The chart is in the form of two bar charts on their sides – the vertical axis (y-axis) represents the group age, while the horizontal axis (x-axis) represents the frequency/proportion of cases [1 - 4].

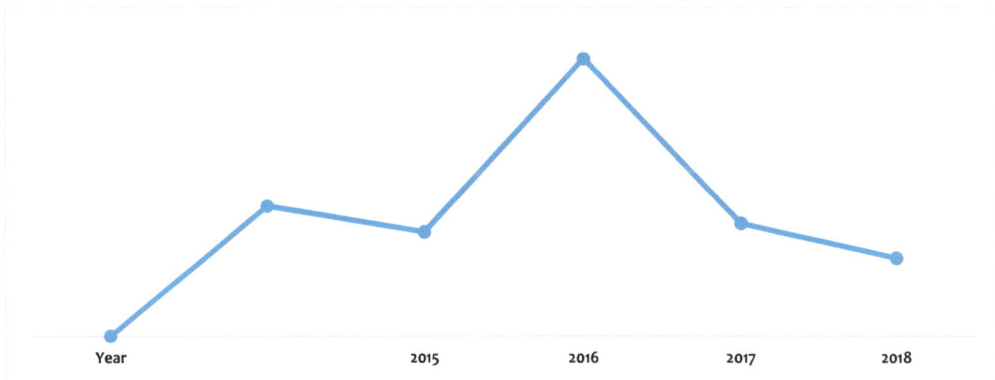

Fig. (6). An example of a line chart of a reported measles in a rural village in country X. (2015-19)

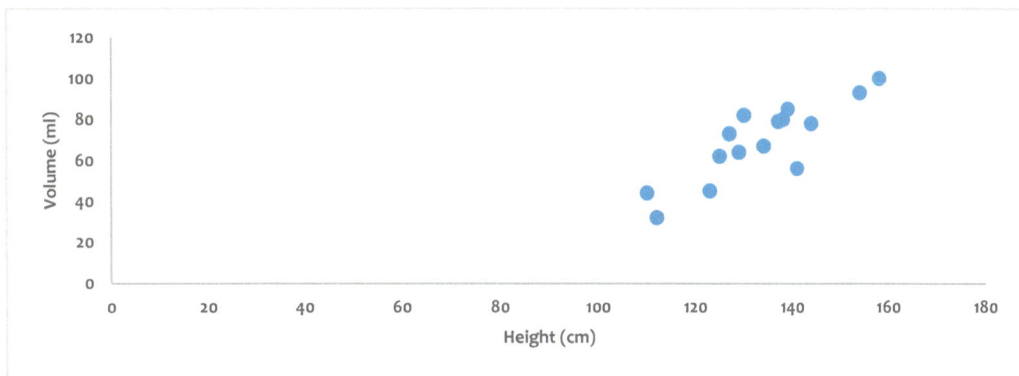

Fig. (7). A scatter plot of men's urine measurements in a study.

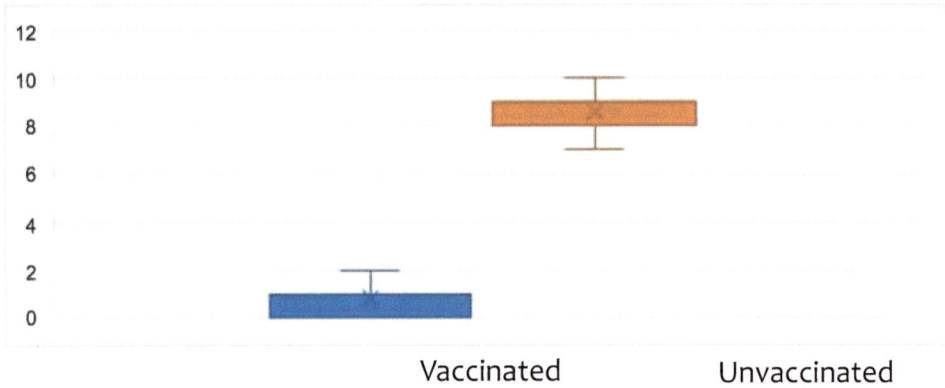

Fig. (8). An example of a 'box' plot showing the incidence of measles in vaccinated and unvaccinated children in a rural community of country X.

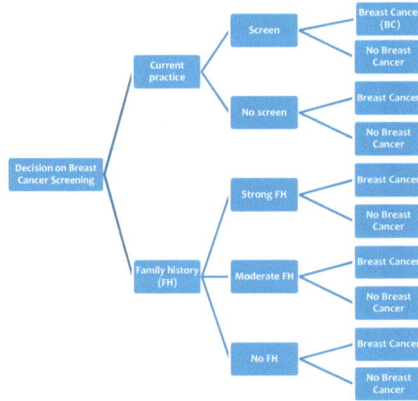

Fig. (9). Decision Tree for Breast Cancer screening in a family.

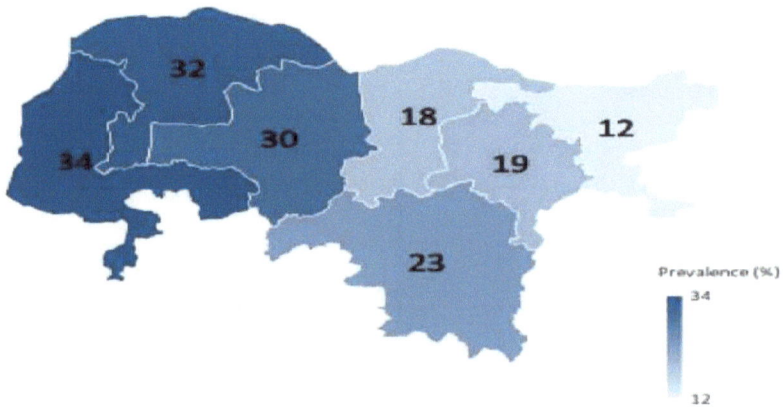

Fig. (10). A map showing an example of hypothetical malaria prevalence during a survey conducted across states in country X in 2015.

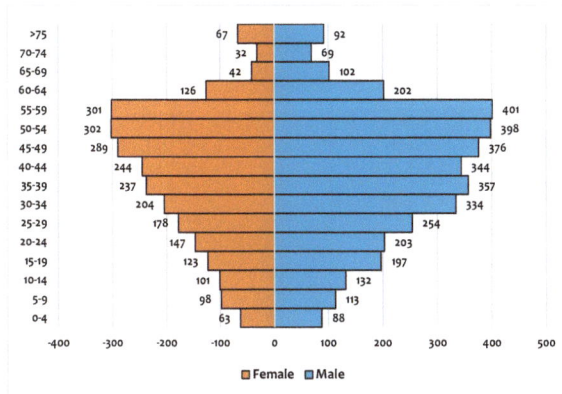

Fig. (11). An example of a population pyramid using data from Table **4**).

Statistical Measure

There are two statistical measures used in epidemiological studies to describe a data set - measures of central tendency (*e.g.*, mode, mean, and median) and measures of dispersion (*e.g.*, range, interquartile range, variance, and standard deviation). In a statistical context, data could either be skewed or normally distributed. It is important to mention that when dealing with normally distributed data, the arithmetic mean is the recommended measure of a central location, and the standard deviation is the recommended measure of spread [1 - 3].

1. Measure of central tendency (or location) is a statistical measurement that quantifies the middle or the centre of a set of distributions and describes where the peak is located. The three most common ways of calculating the location of the central point are the *mode, mean,* and *median*. It is important to note that the *mean* is the most commonly used in statistical computations because of its excellent statistical properties.

The **mode** is the most occurring value in a dataset, and in a small dataset, it is calculated by incrementally arranging the values; the most occurring value is the modal number. When dealing with a large dataset, the values are first arranged into a frequency distribution table. The frequency at which each value occurs is indicated in the adjacent column, and the value with the most frequency is the *mode* (Table).

Example: In a 3-month duration of Hepatitis B vaccination involving 15 people in a workplace, varying doses of the antigen were received by the subjects, as shown below. The mode was calculated as,

Solution: 0, 0, 0, 1, 1, 2, 2, 2, 2, 2, 3, 3, 3, 3, 3

The modal number is 3 because more people received 3 doses of the antigen.

NB: In a distribution, we can have no *mode* if no values appear more than once or more than one mode if two or more values tie as the most frequent. Similarly, the *mode* is not affected by outliers (*i.e.*, one or two extreme values), and, as such, it is a good descriptive measure.

The **median** is the middle value in a dataset after all measurements have been put in ranking order. In simpler terms, when the values are ranked from the smallest to the highest, the value that divides the data into two halves (*i.e.*, one-half of the values is smaller than the *median* value, and the other half is larger) is the statistical *median*. It is considered as the 50th percentile of a distribution.

To find the middle observation in a dataset, use this formula:

Middle position = n +1/2.

Example 1: With odd observation: 2,3,4,5,6, the median is 4.

Solution: Using the formula 5+1/2 = 3. Thus, the 3rd observation is the median, which is 4.

Example 2: With even observation: 2,3,4,5,6,7, the median is 4+5/2 = 4.5.

Solution: Using the formula, 6+1/2 = 3.5. Thus, the median fall between the 3rd and 4th observations, which is 4+5/2 = 4.5

NB: In a distribution, a median can be a single observation or double observation, depending on the dataset. If the middle observations fall within two observations, the median is the average. Similarly, the median is also not affected by outliers (*i.e.*, one or two extreme values) and is a good descriptive measure for **skewed** data.

The **arithmetic mean**, commonly referred to as sample average or mean, is the value that is closest to the other values in a distribution. It is calculated by summing up all values in a distribution and dividing the sum by the number of observations.

Example: Find the mean of this dataset 1, 2, 3, 4, 5, 6, 7, 8, 9, 10

Solution: $(1 + 2 + 3 + 4 + 5 + 6 + 7 + 8 + 9 + 10)/10$

$55/10 = 5.5$

NB: The mean is the centre of the distribution, which is confirmed by subtracting the mean from each observation in the dataset; the sum of the differences will be zero. The mean is the best descriptive measure for *normally* distributed data (not skewed) and is thus affected by outliers (extreme values).

*2. **Measure of spread (dispersion)*** measures the distribution of observations from its central value. It describes the variation of values from that peak in the distribution; the most common is the range, interquartile range, variance, and standard deviation [1 - 3].

The *range* is the difference between the largest and smallest values of a data set. To calculate the range, subtract the minimum from the maximum value.

Example: If the incubation period of COVID-19 patients is 2, 5, 9, 10, 14, the range could be calculated as:

Solution: Range = Maximum value − Minimum value = 14 − 2 = 12

The range is epidemiological as two numbers, *i.e.*, the minimum value to the maximum value (*e.g.*, 12 − 14). However, in a statistical context, the range is reported as a single number, *i.e.*, the difference between the maximum and minimum values (*e.g.*, 12).

To discuss the ***interquartile range***, let us look at percentiles and quartiles. The *percentile* is a value on a scale of 100 that divides the data into 100 equal parts. It indicates a P percent of the observations falling at or below it. In a set of observations, the maximum percentile is 100, and the median value is the 50th percentile. In the case of ***quartiles***, the data could be divided into four equal parts – 25th as the first quartile, 50th as the second quartile, 75th as the third quartile, and 100th as the fourth quartile.

The ***interquartile range***, most commonly used with the median (the 50th percentile), especially when the data are skewed, represents the central portion of the distribution. It includes the second and third quartiles of distribution and, thus, ranges from the 25th to the 75th percentiles.

Step 1: Arrange the data in ascending order. *e.g.*, 0, 2, 7, 9, 10, 12, 14, 18, 19, 22

Step 2: Find the positions for the 1st and 3rd quartiles.

Q1 position = (n+1)/4 = (10+1)/4 = 2.75

Q2 position = 3(n+1)/4 = 3*(10+1)/4 = 8.25

Step 3: Identify the values of 1st quartile (Q1) and 3rd quartile (Q3)

Value of Q1 is the second observation plus ¾ of the difference between the 2nd and 3rd observations = 2 + ¾ (7-2) = 2 + ¾ (5) = 5.75

Value of Q3 is eight observations plus ¼ of the difference between the 8th and 9th observations = 18 + ¼ (19-8) = 18 + ¼ (1) = 18.25

Step 4: Calculate the interquartile range *i.e.*, Q3 − Q1 = 18.25 − 5.75 = 12.5

NB: 1. In the data, the median is 11. To know whether the data are skewed, we should look at the difference between Q1 and the median (11 − 5.75 = 5.25) and Q3 and the median (18.25 − 11 = 7.25).

2. The interquartile ranges (Q1 and Q3) are used with the minimum and maximum values to make a meaningful inference regarding the centre, spread, and shape of the distribution (*i.e.*, minimum value 0, maximum value 22, median 11, Q1 5.75, and Q3 18.25).

The **standard deviation (SD)** is the most widely used measure of spread. When reporting the SD, means should always be reported. It is calculated using the steps as follows:

• Calculating the Arithmetic Mean
• Subtracting the Arithmetic Mean from each value in the observations.
• Squaring the difference in step 2 and summing them up.
• Calculating the Variance by dividing the sum of the squared difference and dividing by (n − 1)
• Considering the SD as the square root of the variance.

Example: In a study to find the mean of the incubation period for COVID-19 virus in 8 subjects, the following number of days were obtained: 2, 4, 6, 8, 3, 12, 14, 15. Using the followng record, the standard deviation was found.

Solution:

AM ($\bar{x}$) = (2 + 4 + 6 + 8 + 3 + 12 + 14 + 15)/8 = 64/8 = 8

Incubation Period (days) x	Mean ($\bar{x}$)	x - $\bar{x}$	(x - $\bar{x}$)2
2	8	-6	36
4	8	-4	16
6	8	-2	4

(Table) cont.....

8	8	0	0
3	8	-5	25
12	8	4	16
14	8	6	36
15	8	7	49
	-	-	182

Variance = $\sum (x - \bar{x})2$ /n-1 = 182/7 = 26 SD = $\sqrt{26}$ = 5.1 days

The ***standard error of the mean (SE)*** is a measure that describes the variability in a distribution from the same population. It assumes that the given data are a sample from a larger population. The standard error quantifies the variation in a set of sample means. It assumes that the mean of each sample is one of an infinite number of the other sample means. It is calculated as follows:

- Calculating the SD
- Dividing the SD by the square root of the number of observations (n)
- Considering the SD as the square root of the value obtained in step 4.

SE = SD/$\sqrt{n}$

Using the SD calculated earlier,

SD = 5.1

SE = SD/$\sqrt{n}$ = 5.1/2.8 = 1.82

Statistical Inference

In epidemiologic research, drawing conclusions beyond the observed data is critical, and this can be done by using a sample to make inferences about the study population. This process is what statisticians refer to as statistical inference. Therefore, statistical inference is important in epidemiology because it enables data to be analyzed effectively to interpret research findings and make meaningful conclusions [8].

In chapter two, we describe that the descriptive studies deal with the properties of the observed data and have no underpinnings to the assumption that the data came from a larger population. In contrast, inferential studies assume that the observed data set is sampled from a larger population. Thus, statistical inference is the process of using data analysis to deduce the properties of an underlying probability distribution. It helps epidemiologists to assess the relationships between the dependent and independent variables [12]. The commonly used statistical inferences that allow researchers to make conclusions include:

1. Confidence Interval

2. Hypothesis testing

3. Correlation Analysis

4. Regression Analysis

5. Chi-square statistics (and contingency table)

6. ANOVA or T-test

The ***Confidence Interval (CI)*** is used by epidemiologists, although not in all epidemiologic measures, to indicate the precision of a measurement. The CI is simply a guide to the variability in a study rather than a strict range of values. It is interpreted as the narrower the CI, the higher the precision. The CI is often used in the following epidemiologic measures: mean, geometric mean, proportions, risk ratio, rate, and odds ratio [1, 2, 12]. In research studies, investigators often set the confidence level at 95% to give them a greater level of confidence, and it is calculated as follows:

- Calculate the mean and its SE
- Multiply the SE by 1.96
- Calculate the lower limit of 95% CI as arithmetic mean – 1.96 x SE
- Calculate the upper limit of the 95% CI as arithmetic mean + 1.96 x SE

Using the worked example for SD and SE above,

Arithmetic Mean = 8 and Standard Error = 1.82

CI = 1.82 x 1.96 = 3.49

Thus,

the lower limit for the 95% CI = 8 – 1.96 x 1.82 = 8 – 3.57 = 4.43

the upper limit for the 95% CI = 8 + 1.96 x 1.82 = 8 + 3.57 = 11.57

Therefore, the CI is 4.4 to 11.6.

From the above example, the best estimate of the true population mean is 8, with the values ranging from 4.4 to 11.6. The CI is narrow, which implies that the sample mean is precise.

It is also critical to note that not every measure of central location and dispersion is well suited for every set of data because observed data rarely approach this ideal normal distribution.

Guide to interpreting CI: If a measurement falls outside of the interval 2 to 15, and the 95% CI is 4.4 to 11.6, it is unlikely that the population mean (μ) is, for example, 17 (it could be if the interval is of the 5% and not 95%). However, there is little risk if one says that the population mean $\neq$ 17. Similarly, scientists can use a CI for hypothesis testing, *e.g.*, $\mu = 17$. This hypothesis is testable, and the result will be to reject it because the CI is 4.4 to 11.6 [1, 2].

Hypotheses *(H)* are statistical assumptions in a statement about an observation that allows it to be tested or refuted. Two types of hypotheses determine whether an exposure is associated or not associated with a health event of interest. Using a descriptive approach, epidemiologists look at the patterns among cases in a given population using time, place, and people to generate hypotheses, aiming to understand the causes and factors behind them [1, 2, 12]. Similarly, through an analytic approach, epidemiologists quantify the level of association between exposure and outcomes to test hypotheses about causal relationships. Generally speaking, and within the context of epidemiologic studies, a **p-*value*** of 0.05 or 5% is used when testing a hypothesis. It is defined as the probability of observing an association between two variables if the null hypothesis is true. It is used in statistical testing to estimate the plausibility of the null hypothesis (*i.e.*, to know if an observed association or difference occurred by chance). In a statistical context, if the *p*-value is smaller than the cutoff point of 0.05, the null hypothesis should be rejected in favour of the alternative hypothesis. These are the null (Ho) and alternative (Ha) hypotheses.

- ***The Null Hypothesis*** *(Ho)* assumes that two (or more) groups do not differ in the measure of interest (*e.g.*, incidence or proportion exposed). It is used in conjunction with statistical testing and assumes that an exposure is not associated with the health event of interest (*i.e.*, risk ratio or odds ratio equals 1).
- ***The Alternative Hypothesis*** *(Ha)* assumes that exposure to a certain agent is associated with a health event of interest. When the null hypothesis proves implausible and is rejected, the alternative hypothesis is accepted.

Correlation (and regression) includes analyses based on multivariate distribution (*i.e.*, a distribution of multiple variables). It describes the strength of an association between two variables (measures their linear association). *Correlation* is a statistical measure determining the presence or absence of an association or relationship between two variables, 'x' and 'y'. The correlation coefficient helps researchers *quantify the extent to which two variables vary together*. If, for example, a researcher deals with two independent variables, it implies that the two values have no relationship (*i.e.*, the variables are not different). However, if the two values are correlated, then the value of the two would be related (*i.e.*, high when the other is either high or low, as the case may be) [2, 13 - 15].

A correlation coefficient denoted as 'r' measures the degree of association. While several tools are used for measuring correlation, the Pearson Correlation Coefficient is the most common. The coefficient, which *measures the linear association between the variables,* ranges between $-1 \leq r \leq 1$, as shown in Figs. (**12a**) to **12d**). When the output is near +1, it is interpreted as there is a strong positive linear association. Conversely, when it is near -1, as shown in Fig. (**12b**), it implies that there is a strong negative association. However, when the value is 0, it implies that there is no linear association, as shown in Fig. **12c**). Correlation is used to ***find a numerical value*** that expresses the relationship between two variables [2].

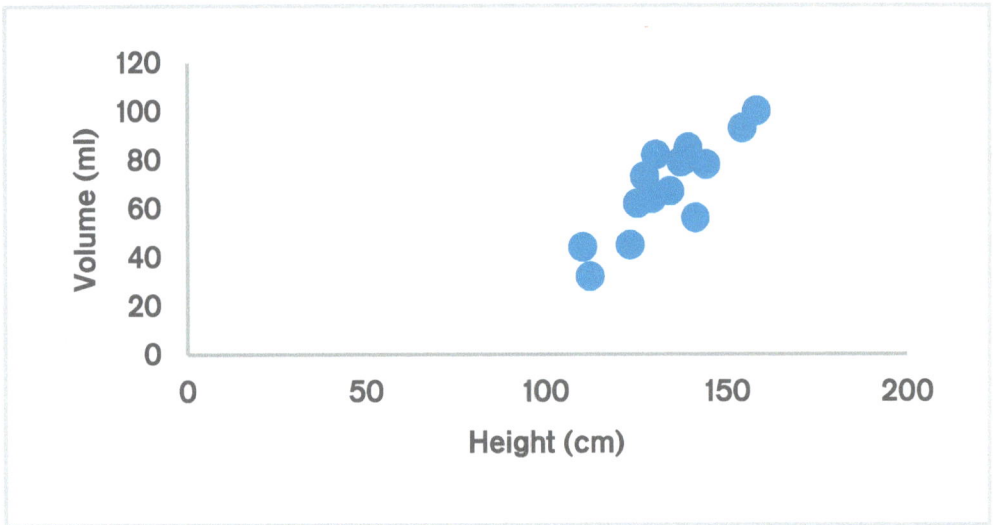

Fig. (12a). The scatter plot of pupil's urine measurement in a study (r = 1).

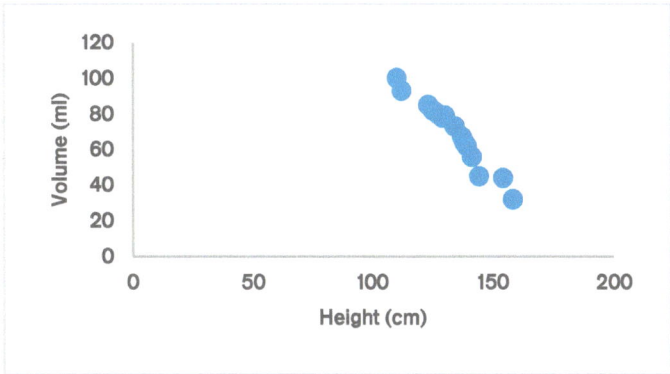

Fig. (12b). The scatter plot of pupil's urine measurement in a study (r = -1).

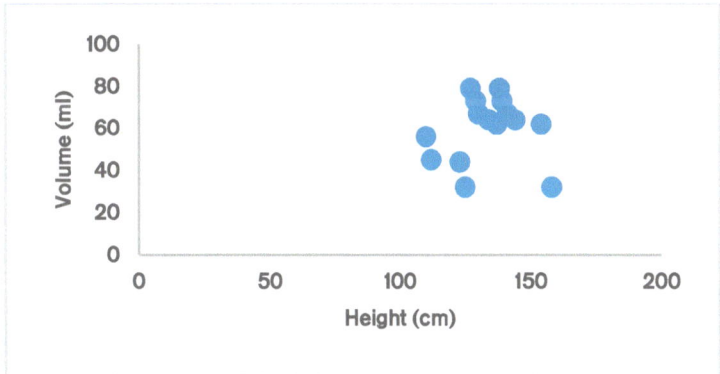

Fig. (12c). The scatter plot of pupil's, urine measurement in a study (r = 0),

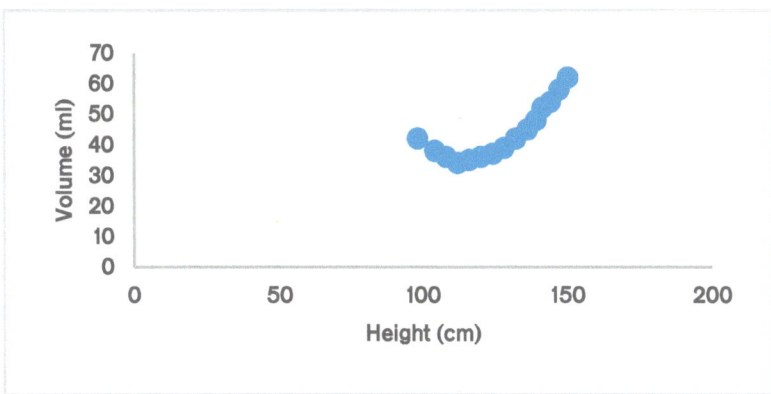

Fig. (12d). The scatter plot of pupil's urine measurement in a study (curved line)

Correlation is calculated as follows:

$$r = \sum (x - \bar{x}) (y - \bar{y}) / \sqrt{[\sum((x - \bar{x})2 (y - \bar{y})2]}$$

Spearman Rank Correlation, Rho $= 1 - (6\sum d2 / n (n2 - 1))$

Regression is an analysis that is based on a multivariate distribution (*i.e.*, a distribution of multiple variables). When there is an association between the two variables (x, y), the relationship can be sought using the regression equation. The regression equation of the changes of y and x could be used in constructing a regression line on a scatter diagram. Regression can be defined as a statistical measure that *predicts the value* of one dependent variable when the value of the independent variable is known [2, 13 - 15]. In a research context, regression analysis helps researchers look at the *impact* of a unit change between the two variables (x, y). The coefficient is the *best-fit line that estimates one variable based on the other variable.* Regression models are considered vital in epidemiological studies. The different types of models are:

- Linear regression (the dependent variable is continuous, and the frequency distribution is normal).
- Logistics regression (the dependent variable is typically represented by 0 or 1)
- Cox proportional hazards (the dependent variable represents the time from a baseline).

Chi-square statistic ($\chi2$) is a statistical test that is used to evaluate the likelihood that the observed frequencies would be based on the assumption that the null hypothesis is true. Thus, a researcher can reject the null hypothesis when the chi-square is greater than 3.84 and *the p*-value is less than 0.05. In statistical research, the data that are used in generating a chi-square statistic must be mutually exclusive and drawn from a large enough sample [2, 13 - 15]. It suffices to say that the chi-square and other similar tests guide researchers in deciding on the null hypothesis.

NB: The Chi-square and similar tests aim to guide researchers in deciding whether to accept or reject the null hypothesis; however, the decision of a researcher could be right or wrong. For example, in a study with fewer participants, a researcher may end up with a *p*-value greater than 0.05 and fail to reject the null hypothesis, while in reality, it is true. Conversely, a study could, by chance, have a *p*-value of less than 0.05.

It is important to mention that the Chi-square statistic is ideal when dealing with a large number of people in a study (preferably more than 30). However, **the Fisher Test** would be ideal when dealing with studies involving fewer participants.

Exposed (A+B) = H1.

Unexposed (C+D) = H0.

Ill (A+C) = I1.

Not ill (B+D) = I2.

Total (T) = 93, H1=48, H0 = 45, I1 = 50, I2 = 43, AD = 1400, BC = 80.

Attack Rate (Risk) is calculated as follows:

In exposed = A/A+B,

In unexposed = C/C+D.

With Ill = I1/T

Using a 2x2 table, as shown in Table 7) , the Chi-square ($\chi2$) can be calculated as follows:

Table 7. Example of Two-by-Two Table.

-	Ill	Not Ill	Total
Exposed	**A (40)**	**B (8)**	**A+B (48)**
Unexposed	C (10)	D (35)	C+D (45)
Total	A+C (50)	B+D (43)	93

T(AD-BC)2/H1*H0*I1*I0

Chi-square = 93(1400 – 80)2 / 48*45*50*43 = 0.93(17424)/464.4 = 34.893.

The Chi-square is 34.893, which is greater than 3.84.

So, the next step is to look up the corresponding value in the Chi-square table; this corresponds to 0.02, which is smaller than the *p*-value of 0.05. Thus, we reject the null hypothesis because the *p*-value is significant (*i.e.*, smaller than 0.05).

NB: The number of degrees of freedom is calculated using *df* = (r 1) x (c 1).

"r" is the number of rows and "c" is the number of columns.

The *Analysis of Variance (ANOVA)* (and the *T-test*) entails hypothesis testing statistical analyses used in epidemiologic studies examining whether the two sample means sufficiently differ. The ANOVA compares more than two sample means; however, when it is used to compare only two sample means, it is similar to running a t-test (NB: the t-test, under the null hypothesis, compares two means of independent samples whether they significantly differ) [2, 13 - 15]. Similarly, ANCOVA (analysis of covariance) includes the covariates during the analysis.

ANOVA is considered a parametric test because it assumes that the populations involved in the study have a normal distribution [14]. As ANOVA compares the variance (or variation) between the data samples, if the variations are much larger, the means of the different samples will not be the same [2, 13 - 15]. As shown below, there are assumptions to consider when running the ANOVA test:

  i. The populations have a normal distribution.
  ii. The populations have the same standard deviation (variance).
iii. The randomly selected samples are independent of each other.

The steps involved in calculating the F value in ANOVA are as follows:

- State the hypotheses (null and alternative, *e.g.*, Ho: $\mu1 = \mu2 = \mu3$, Ha: $\mu1 \neq \mu2 \neq \mu3$)
- State the α level of significance (*e.g.*, 5%)
- Calculate the test statistics in ANOVA,
- Calculate the critical value,
- State decision rule (to accept or reject the null hypothesis)
- Interpret the findings.

Mathematical Modelling

Mathematical models are tools used to study the mechanisms of disease spread, gain insight into the course of the outbreak, and evaluate strategies for the control of the epidemic [17].

Mathematical models, using basic assumptions or collected statistics, are widely used by epidemiologists to project how infectious diseases will progress to prevent an epidemic from happening through instituting public health measures. The models find parameters for the disease under study to compute the effects of various interventions (*e.g.*, mass, drug administration, immunization, *etc.*) [17, 18]. There are two types of epidemic models:

i. ***Stochastic model:*** A stochastic modelling tool estimates the probability distributions of potential outcomes. The model uses variance in risk of exposure within the dynamics of disease and other illnesses.

ii. ***Deterministic model:*** In a deterministic model, we assign individuals in the population to different subgroups or compartments. It uses letters such as S, I, R, M, and E to represent different stages of an epidemic and assign the individuals to the various stages.

While various models are used in epidemics, the SIR model is the most basic. The SIR model uses three compartments: S = susceptible, I = Infected, and R = recovered. There are various statistical applications used for calculating mathematical models.

Similarly, it is critical to mention the ***Reproduction Number (R)*** [20, 21]. The reproduction number could be R, nought, or zero (Ro) or the effective reproduction number (Re). The Ro measures how many people an infected person can infect on average in the absence of preexisting immunity within the community during his infection. Similarly, Re is the number of susceptible people infected by an individual at a given time. The Re changes as people die or with changes in the immunity level of the population, either as a result of immunity from vaccination or infection.

The reproduction rate guides epidemiologists to know whether the infection will spread ($R0 > 1$ means infected person infects more than one other person, $R0 < 1$ means infected person infects less than one person or the epidemic will die out; and $R0 = 1$, means one infected person infects one other person the implication of which is that the disease will remain in the population at endemic level, or the spread of the epidemic will continue).

Assumption Testing

Assumption testing is a critical step in statistical analysis to ensure the validity of the results. Many statistical methods rely on certain assumptions about the data, and if these assumptions are not met, the results can be misleading. The types of assumptions, testing assumptions, and addressing violations are briefly discussed below [2, 13 - 15]:

Types of Assumptions

1. **Normality**: Many statistical tests, such as t-tests and ANOVA, assume that the data follows a normal distribution. To check this assumption, researchers can use graphical methods like Q-Q plots or statistical tests like the Shapiro-Wilk test.

2. **Homogeneity of Variances**: Tests like ANOVA assume that the variances across groups are equal. The Levene's test is commonly used to assess the equality of variances.

3. **Independence**: Statistical tests assume that observations are independent of each other. This assumption is crucial, especially in time-series data or clustered data. Researchers should carefully design studies to ensure independence or use methods that account for dependency.

4. **Linearity**: Regression analysis assumes a linear relationship between the independent and dependent variables. Residual plots can help assess whether this assumption is met.

5. **Absence of Multicollinearity**: In multiple regression, it is assumed that the independent variables are not highly correlated with each other. The Variance Inflation Factor (VIF) is used to detect multicollinearity.

Testing Assumptions

• **Normality**: The Shapiro-Wilk test or Kolmogorov-Smirnov test can be used to test if the data are normally distributed. Visual inspections through histograms or Q-Q plots also provide insights.

• **Homogeneity of Variances**: Levene's test or Bartlett's test can be applied to verify if variances are equal across groups.

• **Independence**: Although no formal test exists for independence, study design and the Durbin-Watson statistic in regression models can help assess this assumption.

• **Linearity**: Scatterplots or residual plots are useful in checking the linearity assumption. If the plot shows a random scatter without patterns, the linearity assumption is likely met.

• **Multicollinearity**: Checking the Variance Inflation Factor (VIF) helps to detect multicollinearity. A VIF value exceeding 10 typically indicates a high level of multicollinearity.

Addressing Violations

If assumptions are violated, researchers may need to apply transformations to the data, use non-parametric tests, or apply different statistical models that are robust to such violations. For example, if the normality assumption is violated, non-parametric tests like the Mann-Whitney U test may be more appropriate than a t-test.

In summary, assumption testing is crucial to ensure the robustness and validity of statistical analysis. By carefully checking and addressing assumptions, researchers can make more accurate and reliable inferences from their data.

CONCLUSION

In conclusion, Chapter 5 has offered a comprehensive overview of statistical methods essential for epidemiological research and practice. By examining fundamental concepts and tools, statistical measures, inference techniques, and mathematical modelling approaches, readers have gained valuable insights into the diverse methodologies employed in data analysis. Moreover, the chapter underscores the importance of sound statistical analysis in informing public health decisions and interventions. As readers progress through subsequent chapters, they will continue to build upon these foundational statistical methods, further enhancing their proficiency in epidemiological research and data analysis.

REFERENCES

[1]   Bonita R, Beaglehole R, Kjellström T. Basic epidemiology. 2nd ed., World Health Organ 2006.

[2]   An Introduction to Applied Epidemiology and Biostatistics.Principles of Epidemiology in Public Health Practice. 3rd ed. Atlanta, GA: Centers for Disease Control and Prevention 2012; p. 30333.

[3]   Field A. Discovering Statistics Using IBM SPSS Statistics. Sage Publications 2022.

[4]   Tufte ER. The Visual Display of Quantitative Information. 3rd ed., Graphics Press 2022.

[5]   Guest G, Namey EE. Public Health Research Methods. SAGE Publications, Inc 2014.

[6]   Townsend JT. Mathematical psychology: Prospects for the 21st century: A guest editorial. J Math Psychol 2008; 52(5): 269-80.
[http://dx.doi.org/10.1016/j.jmp.2008.05.001] [PMID: 19802342]

[7]   Lee J. Measurement scale. Encyclopedia Britannica. 2022. Avaible from: https://www.britannica.com/topic/measurement-scale

[8]   Upton G, Cook I. Oxford Dictionary of Statistics. OUP 2008.
[http://dx.doi.org/10.1093/acref/9780199541454.001.0001]

[9]   Utts JM. Seeing Through Statistics. 3rd ed. Thomson Brooks/Cole 2005; pp. 166-7.

[10]   Wilkinson L. The Grammar of Graphics. 2nd ed., Springer 2020.

[11]   Kamiński B, Jakubczyk M, Szufel P. A framework for sensitivity analysis of decision trees. Cent Eur J Oper Res 2018; 26(1): 135-59.
[http://dx.doi.org/10.1007/s10100-017-0479-6] [PMID: 29375266]

[12]   Tyagi A, Morris J. Using decision analytic methods to assess the utility of family history tools. Am J Prev Med 2003; 24(2): 199-207.
[http://dx.doi.org/10.1016/S0749-3797(02)00594-9] [PMID: 12568827]

[13]   Laake P, Fagerland MW. Statistical Inference.Research in Medical and Biological Sciences. 2nd ed., Academic Press 2015.
[http://dx.doi.org/10.1016/B978-0-12-799943-2.00011-2]

[14]   Vieira S, Corrente JE. Statistical methods for assessing agreement between double readings of clinical measurements. J Appl Oral Sci 2011; 19(5): 488-92.
[http://dx.doi.org/10.1590/S1678-77572011000500009] [PMID: 21986654]

[15]   Peck R, Olsen C, Devore JL. Cengage Learning. 5th ed., 2016.

[16]   Armitage P, Berry G, Matthews JNS. Statistical Methods in Medical Research. 4th ed., Wiley 2001.

[17]   Saleh JEA, Saddiq A, Uchenna AA. LLIN Ownership, Utilization, and Malaria Prevalence: An Outlook at the 2015 Nigeria Malaria Indicator Survey. OAlib 2018; 5(1): 1-12.
[http://dx.doi.org/10.4236/oalib.1104280]

[18]   Daley DJ, Gani J. Epidemic Modeling: An Introduction. NY: Cambridge University Press 2005.

[19]   Brauer F, Castillo-Chávez C. Mathematical Models in Population Biology and Epidemiology. NY: Springer 2001.
[http://dx.doi.org/10.1007/978-1-4757-3516-1]

[20]   van den Driessche P. Reproduction numbers of infectious disease models. Infect Dis Model 2017; 2(3): 288-303.
[http://dx.doi.org/10.1016/j.idm.2017.06.002] [PMID: 29928743]

[21]   Nishiura H, Chowell G. The Effective Reproduction Number as a Prelude to Statistical Estimation of Time-Dependent Epidemic Trends.Mathematical and Statistical Estimation Approaches in Epidemiology. Dordrecht: Springer 2009.
[http://dx.doi.org/10.1007/978-90-481-2313-1_5]

Advanced Epidemiological Methods

Abstract: Chapter 6 delves into sophisticated techniques and approaches shaping contemporary epidemiological research. Beginning with an introduction to the themes of the chapter, it explores advanced statistical techniques that enhance the analysis of complex epidemiological data. The chapter also discusses the integration of genomics into epidemiological studies, illuminating the insights gained and challenges posed by the genomic era. Furthermore, it examines emerging challenges and opportunities in epidemiology, offering perspectives on navigating evolving trends and harnessing novel methodologies to address contemporary public health concerns.

Keywords: Advanced Epidemiological Methods, Data Analysis, Emerging Challenges, Genomics, Opportunities, Public Health, Statistical Techniques.

INTRODUCTION

In our expedition, through the captivating terrain of epidemiology, we have ventured deep into the heart of the discipline, unravelling its history, exploring models, dissecting research designs, and mastering the art of statistical analysis. Now, as we continue our ascent to the summit of epidemiological knowledge, we arrive at a realm where the boundaries of traditional methodology blur, where innovation and sophistication reign supreme—Chapter 6, where the cutting-edge techniques of Advanced Epidemiological Methods await.

Advanced epidemiological methods are the frontier of disease investigation, where complexity meets ingenuity. In this chapter, we embark on an exhilarating journey through the world of techniques and approaches that transcend conventional boundaries, enabling epidemiologists to tackle some of the most intricate and pressing challenges of our time.

This chapter begins by delving into spatial epidemiology, where geography meets epidemiology. It explores how geographic information systems (GIS), satellite imagery, and spatial statistical techniques are harnessed to elucidate the spatial distribution of diseases, identify hotspots, and inform targeted interventions [1, 2]. Through captivating examples, we will witness how spatial epidemiology has

Jalal-Eddeen Abubakar Saleh

revolutionized our understanding of diseases with spatial patterns, from infectious diseases like malaria to chronic conditions like cancer.

Next, we navigate the complex currents of molecular epidemiology, a realm where the genetic code intertwines with disease dynamics. We will uncover how advances in genomics and molecular biology have unlocked the potential to trace the origins of pathogens, unravel transmission networks, and personalize treatment strategies. Molecular epidemiology is at the forefront of our battle against emerging infectious diseases, enabling us to anticipate and respond to new threats with unprecedented precision.

As we proceed, we will explore the art of causal inference—a critical pillar of epidemiology that seeks to establish cause-and-effect relationships amidst the noise of observational data. Through counterfactual frameworks, causal diagrams, and advanced statistical techniques, we will uncover the strategies employed by epidemiologists to decipher the causal pathways that underlie diseases, helping to guide public health interventions with greater confidence.

In the age of digital connectivity, epidemiologists have an abundance of data sources and analytical tools at their disposal. We will delve into data mining, machine learning, and artificial intelligence, witnessing how these technologies are transforming the landscape of epidemiological research. From predicting disease outbreaks to identifying novel risk factors, the fusion of data science and epidemiology opens new horizons for discovery.

As we embark on this journey in Chapter 6, remember that advanced epidemiological methods are not just the tools of the future—they are the solutions to the challenges of today. These methods empower us to address complex questions, unveil hidden truths, and guide policy decisions with unprecedented clarity. This is where the art of epidemiology meets the cutting edge of science, where innovation and tradition converge to shape our understanding of diseases and the health of populations.

Welcome to a chapter that explores the frontiers of epidemiological inquiry, where Advanced Epidemiological Methods unfold like a treasure trove of knowledge and innovation. This is where the future of public health is being forged, where data, technology, and creativity unite to illuminate the path towards healthier societies.

ADVANCED STATISTICAL TECHNIQUES

The Advanced Statistical Techniques encompass a broad and diverse set of advanced methods and approaches used in statistical analysis to tackle complex data-driven problems. These techniques are typically employed when traditional statistical methods are insufficient to extract meaningful insights or make accurate predictions from the data [1, 2]. Some essential advanced statistical techniques include:

1. *Machine Learning Algorithms:* Machine learning encompasses a wide range of algorithms, including decision trees, random forests, support vector machines, neural networks, and deep learning, which can be used for tasks, such as classification, regression, clustering, and pattern recognition.

2. *Bayesian Statistics:* Bayesian methods are used for probabilistic reasoning and updating beliefs based on new evidence. Bayesian techniques are particularly valuable for problems involving uncertainty and parameter estimation.

3. *Time Series Analysis:* This technique uses data collected over time to model and forecast temporal patterns and trends. Time series analysis is vital in finance, economics, and environmental science.

4. *Survival Analysis:* Survival analysis is used to analyse time-to-event data, such as the time to failure or recovery in medical studies. It accounts for censoring and provides insights into event probabilities over time.

5. *Multivariate Analysis:* Multivariate techniques explore the relationships between multiple variables simultaneously, including techniques like principal component analysis (PCA), factor analysis, and canonical correlation analysis (CCA).

6. *Predictive Modeling:* Predictive modelling involves building statistical models to make predictions or classifications. Techniques like logistic regression, support vector machines, and ensemble methods are commonly used.

7. *Spatial Analysis:* Spatial statistics deals with analysing data distributed in space. It includes spatial autocorrelation, spatial interpolation, and geostatistics, among others.

8. *Experimental Design:* Advanced experimental design methods, such as factorial design and response surface methodology, optimise experiments to gather the most information with the fewest resources.

9. *Data Mining:* Data mining techniques involve discovering patterns, associations, and trends in large datasets. Methods like clustering, association rule mining, and text mining fall under this category.

10. Simulation and Monte Carlo Methods: Monte Carlo simulations are used to estimate complex probabilities and make predictions in situations where analytical solutions are difficult to obtain.

These advanced statistical techniques are essential for solving complex problems in various domains, including finance, healthcare, engineering, and social sciences. Their application often requires a solid understanding of statistics, programming skills, and domain-specific knowledge to choose the most appropriate technique and interpret the results effectively [1, 2]. This section will explore two broad areas:

ADVANCED ANALYTIC METHODS

Epidemiology has evolved to encompass advanced statistical techniques that enable researchers to explore complex relationships and patterns in health data. Advanced analytics are not just tools; they are powerful instruments for unlocking deeper insights. Advanced Analytic Methods refer to sophisticated techniques and approaches used to analyze and gain insights from data, often extending beyond traditional statistical methods. These methods are particularly valuable when dealing with complex datasets, unstructured data, or when seeking deeper and more nuanced understanding [1, 2]. Here are some critical components of advanced analytic methods:

i. ***Machine Learning:*** Machine learning encompasses a wide range of algorithms that enable computers to learn from and make predictions or decisions based on data. It includes supervised learning for classification and regression, unsupervised learning for clustering and dimensionality reduction, and reinforcement learning for decision-making tasks.

ii. ***Deep Learning:*** A subset of machine learning, deep learning, involves neural networks with many layers (deep neural networks). It has achieved remarkable success in tasks, such as image recognition, natural language processing, and speech recognition.

iii. ***Natural Language Processing (NLP):*** NLP techniques are used to analyze and understand human language data. It includes sentiment analysis, language translation, text summarization, and chatbots.

iv. ***Computer Vision:*** Computer vision focuses on teaching computers to interpret and understand visual information from images and videos. It is applied in facial recognition, object detection, and autonomous driving, among other fields.

v. ***Big Data Analytics:*** Advanced methods for processing, managing, and analyzing large and complex datasets often use distributed computing frameworks like Hadoop and Spark.

vi. ***Anomaly Detection:*** Anomaly detection techniques identify unusual patterns or outliers in data. These methods are essential for fraud detection, network security, and quality control.

vii. ***Predictive Analytics:*** Predictive modelling and analytics involve using historical data to predict future events or trends. It is widely applied in forecasting customer retention and resource optimization.

viii. ***Ensemble Methods:*** Ensemble techniques combine multiple models to improve prediction accuracy and robustness. Examples include random forests, gradient boosting, and stacking.

ix. ***Time Series Forecasting:*** Time series analysis and forecasting methods are used to predict future values in a time-ordered data sequence, which is crucial for demand forecasting and financial prediction.

x. ***Reinforcement Learning:*** A subset of machine learning, reinforcement learning, focuses on training agents to make sequential decisions by interacting with the environment. Applications include game-playing algorithms and autonomous robotics.

xi. ***Bayesian Networks:*** Bayesian networks model probabilistic relationships between variables using directed acyclic graphs. They are helpful for probabilistic reasoning and decision-making under uncertainty.

xii. ***Graph Analytics:*** Graph analytics involves the analysis of complex networks or graphs to uncover patterns and relationships. Applications range from social network analysis to supply chain optimization.

xiii. ***Advanced Visualization:*** Cutting-edge visualization techniques help present complex data understandably and interactively, aiding in data exploration and communication of findings.

Advanced analytic methods often require a strong foundation in mathematics, programming skills, and domain knowledge. They are employed in various industries, including healthcare, finance, marketing, and scientific research, to extract valuable insights, make informed decisions, and gain a competitive edge in data-driven decision-making [1, 2].

SPATIAL AND TEMPORAL ANALYSIS

Spatial Analysis

Involves examining data in relation to its geographic or spatial context. It aims to uncover patterns, relationships, and insights that are influenced by location and spatial attributes. A more in-depth discussion of spatial analysis is given below:

a. ***Geographic Information Systems (GIS):*** GIS is a powerful tool in spatial analysis. It allows for the creation, storage, manipulation, and visualization of geographic data. GIS can be used to map spatial features, perform spatial queries, and analyze the distribution of data points on maps.

b. ***Spatial Patterns***: Spatial analysis helps identify patterns, such as clustering (points or events occurring closely together), dispersion (points or events spread apart), and spatial autocorrelation (the degree of similarity or dissimilarity between neighbouring locations).

c. ***Spatial Interpolation:*** This technique estimates values at unmeasured locations based on values observed at nearby locations. Methods like kriging, inverse distance weighting, and spline interpolation are commonly used to create continuous surfaces from sparse data points.

d. ***Spatial Autocorrelation***: This concept measures the degree to which data values in one location are related to data values in nearby locations. Positive spatial autocorrelation indicates spatial clustering, while negative spatial autocorrelation indicates dispersion.

e. ***Spatial Regression***: Spatial regression models account for spatial dependencies in data. They help analyze how spatial factors influence the dependent variable, making them valuable in economics and epidemiology.

f. ***Spatial Data Visualization***: Visualization tools, including choropleth maps, heat maps, and spatial graphs, help convey spatial patterns and trends effectively.

g. **Map Images:** Incorporating map images can enhance the understanding of spatial patterns. Examples of map images include Disease Incidence Maps (maps showing the distribution of disease cases across regions), Heat Maps (visualizations that highlight areas with higher densities of health events), and Cluster Maps (maps identifying statistically significant clusters of disease cases).

Fig. (**1**) showing an example of classic strata of malaria endemicity [3].

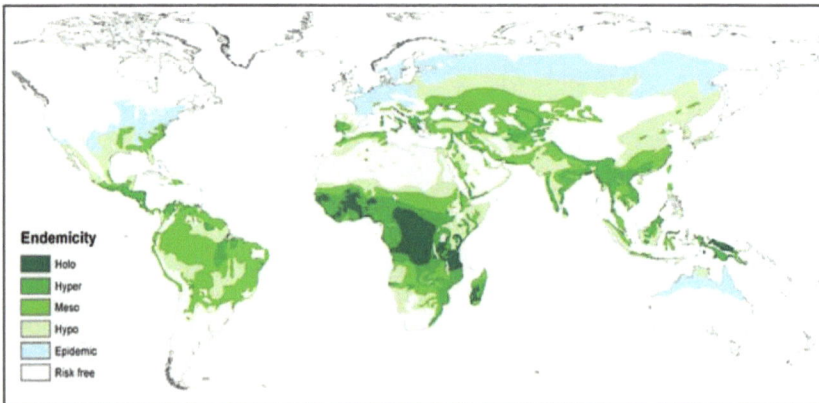

Endemicity
- Holo
- Hyper
- Meso
- Hypo
- Epidemic
- Risk free

Fig. (1). An example of classic strata of malaria endemicity.

Temporal Analysis

Also referred to as time series analysis, focuses on understanding data that varies over time. This type of analysis is essential for making predictions, identifying trends, and making informed decisions based on temporal patterns [1, 2]. A more detailed look at temporal analysis is presented below:

a. ***Time Series Data:*** Time series data is sequential data collected regularly. Examples include stock prices, weather measurements, and daily sales figures.

b. ***Trend Analysis:*** Trend analysis aims to identify long-term patterns or trends in time series data. It helps understand whether a dataset is increasing, decreasing, or stable over time.

c. ***Seasonal Decomposition:*** Seasonal decomposition separates a time series into its trend, seasonal, and residual components. It helps understand periodic patterns, such as yearly or monthly fluctuations.

d. ***Time Series Forecasting:*** Time series forecasting uses historical data to predict future values. Methods include autoregressive integrated moving average (ARIMA), exponential smoothing, and machine learning algorithms like LSTM (Long Short-Term Memory) networks.

e. ***Event Analysis:*** Event analysis involves studying the impact of specific events or interventions on a time series. For instance, how does a marketing campaign affect sales over time?

f. ***Survival Analysis:*** Survival analysis deals with time-to-event data, such as the time to failure of a machine or the time to a specific event. It considers censoring, where some events may not have occurred by the end of the study.

g. ***Temporal Data Mining***: Temporal data mining involves discovering patterns, associations, and anomalies in time-stamped data. It is valuable for understanding customer behaviour, detecting fraud, and optimizing processes.

h. ***Spectral Analysis:*** Spectral analysis examines the frequency components of time series data, revealing periodicity and cyclic behaviour. It is used in fields like signal processing and environmental monitoring.

Both spatial and temporal analysis are vital in various domains, including epidemiology (tracking disease outbreaks), environmental science (studying climate change), finance (forecasting stock prices), and transportation (optimizing routes and schedules). Combining these analyses, known as spatiotemporal analysis, can provide even deeper insights into how data vary across space and time, enabling more informed decision-making and problem-solving [1, 2].

Exercise 1: Applying Advanced Statistical Techniques to Local Health Issues

In this exercise, readers will apply advanced statistical techniques to address local health issues:

   i. **Select a Local Health Issue:** Choose a health problem or issue specific to your region or community. Consider data availability and the potential impact of advanced statistical analysis.

  ii. **Gather Data:** Collect relevant data related to the selected health issue. This could include epidemiological data, demographic information, environmental factors, or any other pertinent variables.

 iii. **Choose the Appropriate Analytic Method:** Based on the nature of your data and research question, select an advanced statistical method from the list provided earlier.

 iv. **Conduct Analysis:** Apply the chosen statistical technique to your dataset. Interpret the results and assess whether there are significant associations or patterns.

  v. **Report Findings:** Prepare a report summarizing your findings, including any implications for public health or policy. Highlight how the advanced statistical analysis adds value to addressing the local health issue.

 vi. **Discussion and Reflection:** Engage in a discussion or reflection on the challenges and advantages of using advanced statistical techniques for local health problems. Consider the potential limitations and future research directions.

This exercise encourages readers to explore the power of advanced statistical techniques in solving complex health problems. It underscores the importance of data-driven decision-making and evidence-based interventions in public health practice.

EPIDEMIOLOGY IN THE GENOMIC ERA

This section will discuss Genomic Epidemiology, Precision Medicine, and Personalized Health. These two are transformative approaches in healthcare that aim to tailor medical decisions, treatments, and interventions to the unique characteristics of each individual.

Genomic Epidemiology

The advent of the genomic era has transformed epidemiology by integrating genomics into the study of disease distribution and determinants. Genomic epidemiology focuses on understanding how genetic variations contribute to disease risk and how genes interact with environmental factors. It is a specialized field that combines genomics, epidemiology, and bioinformatics to understand and combat infectious diseases at a molecular level. It plays a crucial role in tracking the spread of pathogens, investigating disease outbreaks, and developing targeted interventions [4]. An in-depth discussion of genomic epidemiology is given below.

Genomic Epidemiology is a powerful tool that enhances our ability to monitor, understand, and respond to infectious diseases. It bridges the gap between genomics and public health, enabling more precise and timely interventions to mitigate the impact of outbreaks and prevent the spread of pathogens. As technology advances and genomic data becomes more accessible, the field of genomic epidemiology will continue to play a critical role in global health. Genomics Epidemiology uses genomic sequencing and analysis to study the transmission, dynamics, genetic diversity, and evolution of pathogens, particularly viruses and bacteria, in populations [4].

Techniques

i. **Whole Genome Sequencing (WGS):** This technique involves sequencing the entire genome of an organism or pathogen. It provides high-resolution data for detailed genetic analysis.
ii. **Metagenomics:**This technique analyzes genetic material directly from environmental samples or clinical specimens, which can reveal the presence of multiple organisms simultaneously.
iii. **Phylogenetics:** The study of the evolutionary relationships between organisms is based on genetic data, often represented as phylogenetic trees.

Applications of Genomic Epidemiology

i. **Disease Outbreak Investigation**: Genomic epidemiology can rapidly identify the source of outbreaks, trace transmission chains, and differentiate between primary and secondary cases.
ii. **Drug Resistance Monitoring:** It helps monitor the emergence of drug-resistant strains of pathogens and guides treatment strategies.
iii. **Vaccine Development:** By understanding the genetic diversity of pathogens, researchers can design more effective vaccines.
iv. **Molecular Epidemiology:** It provides insights into how pathogens adapt to human populations and evolve over time.
v. **Pathogen Surveillance:** Genomic data can be used for continuous monitoring of pathogen populations to detect emerging threats.

Key Components of Genomic Epidemiology

i. **Data Collection:** Obtaining samples from infected individuals, isolating the pathogen, and conducting genomic sequencing.

ii. **Data Analysis**: Processing and analyzing genomic data to identify genetic variants, mutations, and phylogenetic relationships.

iii. **Interpretation:** Interpreting the genomic data in the context of epidemiological information, such as patient travel history, contacts, and clinical outcomes.

iv. **Visualization:** Creating phylogenetic trees, heatmaps, and other visualizations to communicate findings effectively.

Challenges and Limitations

i. **Data Integration:** Combining genomic data with epidemiological and clinical data can be complex but is crucial for a comprehensive understanding of disease dynamics.

ii. **Sampling Bias:** The selection of samples for sequencing may not always represent the entire population, leading to potential biases.

iii. **Data Privacy:** Handling sensitive patient data requires strict adherence to ethical and privacy standards.

iv. **Resource Constraints:** Genomic sequencing and analysis can be expensive and require specialized equipment and expertise.

v. **Evolutionary Complexity:** Pathogens can rapidly evolve, making it challenging to accurately track and predict their behaviour.

Real-World Examples

i. **COVID-19 Pandemic**: Genomic epidemiology played a pivotal role in tracking the spread of the SARS-CoV-2 virus, identifying new variants, and informing vaccination efforts.

ii. **Ebola Outbreaks:** Genomic analysis has helped trace the sources of Ebola outbreaks in Africa and understand how the virus evolves.

iii. **Antibiotic Resistance:** Researchers use genomics to study the genetic mechanisms behind antibiotic resistance in bacteria like Methicillin-resistant Staphylococcus aureus (MRSA).

Genomic epidemiology forms the basis for precision medicine and personalized health initiatives. Precision medicine aims to provide tailored medical care based on a person's unique genetic and environmental factors [4]. Key aspects include:

a. **Risk Prediction:** Genomic information can enhance risk prediction models, helping identify individuals at higher risk for specific diseases. This allows for early intervention and prevention.

b. **Treatment Optimization:** Personalized treatment plans consider genetic factors to determine the most effective therapies with minimal side effects.

c. **Disease Prevention**: Genomic information can guide preventive measures and lifestyle recommendations to reduce disease risk.

PRECISION MEDICINE AND PERSONALIZED HEALTH

represent a paradigm shift in healthcare, emphasizing individualization and customization of medical care and health promotion. These approaches hold the promise of improving health outcomes, enhancing patient engagement, and revolutionizing healthcare delivery in the years to come [5]. This approach is rooted in the idea that one-size-fits-all healthcare may not be the most effective and that considering genetic, environmental, and lifestyle factors can lead to more precise and personalized medical care [5]. An in-depth exploration of precision medicine and personalized health is presented below:

Precision Medicine

Is also known as personalized medicine. It is an approach to medical care that considers individual variability in genes, environment, and lifestyle. It aims to target the right treatment to the right person at the right time [5].

Key Components

i. **Genomics**: The study of the genetic makeup of an individual, including DNA sequencing and analysis, plays a central role in precision medicine.

ii. **Biomarkers**: Molecular indicators, such as genetic mutations or protein levels, are used to identify disease risk, progression, and treatment response.

iii. **Tailored Treatments:** Treatment plans are customized based on genetic and molecular profiles, optimizing therapeutic outcomes.

Applications

i. **Cancer**: Precision oncology uses genomic information to match cancer patients to targeted therapies, improving response rates and minimizing side effects.

ii. **Pharmacogenomics**: It personalizes drug selection and dosing based on the genetic makeup of an individual, enhancing medication safety and efficacy.

iii. **Rare Diseases:** Precision medicine aids in diagnosing and treating rare genetic disorders by identifying the underlying genetic mutations.

Personalized Health

Encompasses a broader perspective, extending beyond medical treatment to consider the overall well-being of an individual [5]. It integrates health promotion, disease prevention, and healthcare decision-making to align with the unique characteristics of an individual.

Key Components

i. **Preventive Strategies:** Personalized health strategies include tailored lifestyle recommendations, such as diet and exercise plans, based on genetic and environmental factors.
ii. **Behavioral Health:** Mental health support and interventions can be personalized to address specific psychological and emotional needs.
iii. **Patient-Centered Care:** Healthcare providers work in partnership with patients to co-create personalized care plans, considering patient preferences and values.

Applications

i. **Chronic Disease Management**: Personalized health interventions can help manage chronic conditions, such as diabetes, by customizing treatment and self-care plans.
ii. **Wellness and Lifestyle**: Individuals can receive guidance on optimizing their lifestyle choices for improved health, from nutrition to stress management.
iii. **Preventive Screenings:** Personalized health may involve risk assessments and tailored recommendations for preventive screening based on genetic predisposition.

Genomic Information

Advances in DNA sequencing technology have made it more accessible and cost-effective to obtain the genetic information of an individual. Genomic data are analyzed to identify disease-associated genetic variants (mutations) and predict disease risk. Genomic information is integrated into medical practice to guide diagnosis, treatment decisions, and preventive measures [5].

Benefits

i. **Tailored Treatments:** Precision medicine can improve treatment efficacy and reduce adverse effects by matching therapies to an individual's genetic profile.
ii. **Disease Prevention**: Personalized health approaches help identify and mitigate disease risks through targeted interventions.

iii. **Patient Engagement**: Patients become active participants in their healthcare decisions, leading to greater satisfaction and adherence to treatment plans.

Challenges

  i. **Data Privacy:** Protecting the security and privacy of personal genetic data is a critical concern.
 ii. **Equity:** Ensuring that personalized healthcare is accessible and equitable for all populations is a critical concern.
iii. **Evidence-Based Practice**: Ensuring that personalized interventions are based on robust scientific evidence is also a critical concern.

Future Directions

Ongoing advancements in genomics, data analytics, and digital health technologies will continue to expand the scope and impact of precision medicine and personalized health [5]. Collaborative efforts among healthcare providers, researchers, policymakers, and patients will be essential in realizing the full potential of these approaches.

Exercise 2: Exploring Genomic Epidemiology in Your Context

In this exercise, readers will explore genomic epidemiology in their local context:

  i. **Select a Disease of Interest:** Choose a prevalent disease or health issue in your region or community that has a potential genetic component, such as diabetes, cancer, or a genetic disorder.
 ii. **Research Genetic Factors:** Investigate the existing knowledge about genetic factors associated with the selected disease. Look for studies, reports, or genetic data relevant to your region.
iii. **Explore Precision Medicine Initiatives:** Identify any precision medicine or personalized health initiatives in your area. These may involve genetic testing, risk assessment, or tailored treatment strategies.
iv. Interview Experts: If possible, interview experts or healthcare professionals working in the field of genomic epidemiology or precision medicine. Seek insights into local efforts and challenges.
 v. **Reflect on Applications:** Reflect on how genomic epidemiology and precision medicine can benefit your community. Consider the potential barriers and ethical considerations.
vi. **Propose Recommendations:** Based on your research and reflections, propose recommendations for integrating genomic epidemiology and precision medicine into local healthcare or public health programs.

This exercise encourages readers to explore the role of genomic epidemiology and personalized health in addressing health challenges specific to their region. It emphasizes the potential for tailored interventions and the importance of staying informed about advancements in genomics and its applications in healthcare.

EMERGING CHALLENGES AND OPPORTUNITIES IN EPIDEMIOLOGY

This section discusses Environmental Epidemiology, Epidemiology of Non-Communicable Diseases (NCDs), Disease Surveillance, and Global Health and Pandemics.

Environmental Epidemiology

Explores the impact of environmental factors on public health. It investigates how exposures to pollutants, toxins, and other environmental agents contribute to disease. Environmental Epidemiology is a branch of epidemiology that studies how environmental factors impact human health [6]. It aims to understand the relationship between exposure to environmental hazards and the occurrence of diseases or health conditions within populations. It is essential for identifying and addressing environmental health risks, especially in emerging challenges like climate change, air quality, and chemical exposures [6]. It serves as a critical bridge between environmental science and public health, ultimately aiming to improve the well-being of populations by reducing the adverse health effects of environmental hazards. The key areas of focus include:

1. **Air Quality and Respiratory Health**: Studying the health effects of air pollutants, such as particulate matter, ozone, and volatile organic compounds, on respiratory diseases like asthma and chronic obstructive pulmonary disease (COPD).

2. **Waterborne Diseases**: Investigating the role of contaminated water sources in the transmission of diseases like cholera, dysentery, and waterborne infections.

3. **Occupational Health:** Assessing health risks in workplaces and understanding occupational exposures that may lead to occupational diseases or injuries.

Environmental Exposure encompasses a wide range of factors in the external environment that can affect human health. These may include pollutants, toxins, chemicals, radiation, biological agents, and lifestyle factors the environment influences [6].

Examples: Air pollution (*e.g.*, particulate matter and pollutants like nitrogen dioxide), water contaminants (*e.g.*, lead and pathogens), pesticides, radiation (*e.g.*,

UV radiation and ionizing radiation), and lifestyle factors influenced by the environment (*e.g.*, diet and physical activity) are its examples.

Objectives of Environmental Epidemiology

i. *Identify Causation:* Environmental epidemiologists seek to determine whether specific environmental exposures are causally linked to particular health outcomes.

ii. *Assess Risk:*They aim to quantify the risk associated with environmental exposures, including dose-response relationships.

iii. *Inform Policy:*They aim to provide evidence for developing public health policies and regulations to reduce or mitigate environmental hazards.

iv. *Prevent and Control:*The goal is to contribute to preventing and controlling environmentally related diseases.

Methods and Approaches

i. *Study Designs:* Environmental epidemiologists use various study designs, including cohort studies, case-control studies, cross-sectional studies, and ecological studies. Longitudinal cohort studies are often favoured for establishing causation.

ii. *Exposure Assessment:* Precise measurement of environmental exposures is crucial. It may involve environmental monitoring, biomarker assessment, surveys, and geospatial analysis.

iii. **Statistical Analysis**: Statistical techniques are used to analyze data and control for confounding variables, including age, gender, and socioeconomic status.

iv. *Meta-Analysis:* Combining and analyzing results from multiple studies can provide a more comprehensive assessment of the evidence.

Key Concepts and Challenges

i. *Latency Periods:* Some environmental exposures may have long latency periods, making establishing a direct causal link with health outcomes challenging.

ii. *Multiple Exposures:* Individuals are often exposed to a combination of environmental factors, making it difficult to isolate the impact of a single exposure.

iii. *Susceptibility*: Genetic, demographic, and health factors can influence the susceptibility of an individual to environmental hazards.

iv. *Cumulative Effects*: The cumulative impact of repeated or chronic exposures is a critical consideration in environmental epidemiology.

Examples of Environmental Epidemiological Studies

i. *Lead Exposure and Neurodevelopmental Effects*: Studies have demonstrated the adverse effects of lead exposure on the cognitive development of children.

ii. *Air Pollution and Respiratory Disease:* Research has linked air pollutants like fine particulate matter (PM2.5) to respiratory conditions like asthma and bronchitis.

iii. *Pesticide Exposure and Cancer:* Investigations have explored the relationship between pesticide exposure in agricultural settings and cancer risk.

iv. *Ultraviolet (UV) Radiation and Skin Cancer:* Studies have shown a clear association between UV radiation exposure (sunlight) and the development of skin cancer.

Policy Implications

i. *Regulations and Standards:* The findings of environmental epidemiological studies often contribute to developing environmental regulations and safety standards.

ii. *Public Health Interventions*: Insights from environmental epidemiology inform public health interventions, such as clean energy initiatives, water quality improvements, and pollution control measures.

iii. *Environmental Justice:* Environmental epidemiology plays a role in advocating for an equitable distribution of environmental benefits and burdens, addressing environmental disparities among communities.

Epidemiology of Non-Communicable Diseases (NCDs)

Such as diabetes, hypertension, and cancer, are a major public health concern. Understanding the epidemiology of these diseases requires an examination of the interactions between agents, hosts, and environments [7].

- **Diabetes:**
- **Agent:** The primary agents include genetic predispositions and lifestyle factors, such as diet and physical activity.
- **Host**: Individuals with a family history of diabetes, obesity, and a sedentary lifestyle are at higher risk.
- **Environment:** Urbanization, poor diet, and lack of access to healthcare services contribute to diabetes prevalence.
- **Hypertension:**
- **Agent**: Risk factors include high salt intake, obesity, and genetic predispositions.
- **Host**: People with a family history of hypertension, older adults, and those with

unhealthy lifestyles are more vulnerable.
- **Environment**: Stressful environments, urban living, and limited access to healthcare can exacerbate hypertension.
- **Cancer**:
- **Agent**: Carcinogens, including tobacco smoke, environmental pollutants, and certain infections, contribute to cancer risk.
- **Host**: Genetic mutations, family history, and personal behaviours (*e.g.*, smoking) are significant risk factors.
- **Environment**: Environmental exposures, such as pollutants and occupational hazards, play a crucial role in cancer epidemiology.

Disease Surveillance

Involves systematically collecting, analyzing, and interpreting health data to monitor and respond to disease outbreaks and trends. In the modern era, technological advancements have transformed surveillance methods [8].

Modern Surveillance Techniques

- **Electronic Health Records (EHRs):** EHRs facilitate real-time data collection and analysis, improving the accuracy and timeliness of disease reporting.
- **Mobile Health Apps:** Apps that track health data and symptoms can provide valuable insights into disease patterns and public health needs.
- **Big Data Analytics**: Advanced analytics and machine learning algorithms can process vast amounts of data from diverse sources to identify trends and predict outbreaks.
- **Challenges and Opportunities:**
- **Data Integration:** Combining data from various sources (*e.g.*, EHRs, social media) can enhance surveillance but also poses challenges related to data quality and privacy.
- **Real-Time Monitoring:** The ability to conduct real-time surveillance improves response times but requires robust infrastructure and data management systems.

Global Health and Pandemics

The field of epidemiology extends beyond local and national borders, addressing global health challenges and pandemic threats. Global Health and pandemics is a critical field encompassing various aspects, including infectious disease surveillance, vaccine epidemiology, and the One Health approach [9]. These components are vital in understanding, monitoring, and responding to infectious disease threats at a global scale. The focus would be on three areas - *Infectious Diseases Surveillance, Vaccine Epidemiology and One Health Approach*:

i. Infectious Disease Surveillance involves systematic data collection, analysis, interpretation, and dissemination of information related to infectious diseases to guide public health action. It involves monitoring the emergence and spread of infectious diseases on a global scale, including efforts to control pandemics like COVID-19 [9].

Key Objectives

- ***Early Detection***: Surveillance systems aim to identify outbreaks and epidemics as early as possible, allowing for prompt response.
- ***Monitoring Trends:*** They track disease trends, including geographic distribution, incidence rates, and changes in pathogen characteristics.
- ***Assessment of Interventions***: Surveillance data help assess the impact of interventions, such as vaccination campaigns or public health measures.

Methods and Tools

- ***Case Reporting***: Healthcare providers report cases of notifiable diseases to public health authorities.
- ***Laboratory Testing:*** Laboratory testing of samples helps confirm diagnosis and identify specific pathogens.
- ***Syndromic Surveillance:*** Monitoring patterns of symptoms or syndromes can provide early indicators of outbreaks.
- ***Electronic Health Records (EHRs):*** EHRs can facilitate real-time data sharing between healthcare facilities.

Global Surveillance Networks

- The World Health Organization (WHO) operates the Global Outbreak Alert and Response Network (GOARN) to facilitate global disease surveillance and response.
- The Centers for Disease Control and Prevention (CDC) in the United States operates the Epidemic Intelligence Service (EIS), a renowned training program for epidemiologists specializing in outbreak investigation.
    - i. ***Vaccine Epidemiology*** is the study of vaccines and their impact on population health. It focuses on vaccine effectiveness, safety, coverage, and evaluation of vaccination programs. It helps in evaluating the effectiveness of vaccination programs in preventing infectious diseases and achieving herd immunity [9].

Key Concepts

- ***Vaccine Effectiveness***: It measures the degree to which a vaccine reduces the incidence of disease in vaccinated populations under real-world conditions.

- *Herd Immunity*: It involves the level of vaccination coverage required to protect a community from an infectious disease outbreak by reducing the transmission of the pathogen.
- *Vaccine Safety:*It monitors adverse events following immunization (AEFI) to ensure the safety of vaccines.

- *Vaccine Coverage:* It assesses the proportion of the population vaccinated against specific diseases.

Importance in Pandemics

- During pandemics, vaccines play a crucial role in controlling the spread of infectious diseases and mitigating their impact.
- Vaccine epidemiology helps guide vaccine distribution strategies, prioritizing vulnerable populations and assessing the impact of vaccination campaigns.
  - i. **One Health Approach** recognizes the interconnectedness of human, animal, and environmental health. It emphasizes collaboration across multiple disciplines to address health threats at the interface of humans, animals, and ecosystems. It recognizes the interconnectedness of human, animal, and environmental health and its relevance in preventing zoonotic disease outbreaks [9].

Key Principles

- *Interdisciplinary Collaboration:* Bringing together experts from human health, veterinary medicine, environmental science, and other fields.
- *Holistic Perspective:* Recognizing that health issues in one sector can have ripple effects across others.
- *Prevention and Preparedness:* Emphasizing proactive measures to prevent disease emergence and spread.

Relevance to Pandemics

- Many infectious diseases that lead to pandemics, such as zoonotic diseases (*e.g.*, COVID-19, H1N1 influenza), originate in animals.
- One Health approach is crucial for the early detection, monitoring, and control of emerging infectious diseases, as it considers the ecological and behavioural factors driving disease transmission.

Global Health and Pandemics encompass a multifaceted approach to addressing infectious disease threats at a global scale. Infectious disease surveillance provides the foundation for early detection and response, vaccine epidemiology guides vaccination strategies, and the One Health approach recognizes the interconnectedness of human, animal, and environmental health. Together, these components play a critical role in preventing, preparing for, and responding to pandemics, ensuring the health and well-being of populations worldwide [9].

Exercise 3: Addressing Environmental Health Issues in Your Region

In this exercise, readers will explore environmental health issues in their region and propose strategies for addressing them:

   i. **Identify Environmental Health Concerns:** Research and identify prevalent environmental health issues in your community or region. These may include air pollution, water contamination, industrial waste, or other environmental hazards.

   ii. **Collect Local Data:** Gather data or reports related to environmental health concerns. This could include air quality monitoring data, water quality reports, or health statistics.

   iii. **Assess Health Impact:** Evaluate the potential health impact of the identified environmental issues. Consider the diseases or health conditions associated with these exposures.

   iv. **Propose Mitigation Strategies**: Develop a list of strategies to mitigate or address environmental health concerns. These may include policy recommendations, community education initiatives, or environmental regulations.

   v. **Engage Stakeholders:** Identify relevant stakeholders, including government agencies, local organizations, and community leaders, and consider how to involve them in addressing the issues.

   vi. **Create an Action Plan**: Outline an action plan for implementing your proposed strategy. Consider timelines, resource requirements, and key responsible parties.

   vii. **Reflect on Challenges and Benefits:** Reflect on the potential challenges and benefits of addressing environmental health issues in your region. Consider the long-term impact on public health.

This exercise encourages readers to engage with pressing environmental health challenges in their local context. It highlights the role of epidemiology in identifying and addressing environmental health concerns, ultimately contributing to healthier communities.

CONCLUSION

In conclusion, Chapter 6 has provided a comprehensive overview of advanced epidemiological methods, encompassing advanced statistical techniques, genomics, and emerging challenges and opportunities in the field. By exploring sophisticated methodologies and emerging trends, readers have gained valuable insights into contemporary approaches to epidemiological research and practice. Moreover, the chapter underscores the importance of embracing innovation and adaptability in addressing evolving public health concerns. As readers continue to engage with subsequent chapters, they will further deepen their understanding of advanced epidemiological methods and their applications in addressing complex health challenges.

REFERENCES

[1]   Rothman KJ, Greenland S, Lash TL. Modern Epidemiology. 3rd ed., Lippincott Williams & Wilkins 2008.

[2]   Elliott P, Wartenberg D, Wakefield J. Spatial epidemiology: Current approaches and future challenges. Environ Health Perspect 2000; 108 (Suppl. 1): 11-9.
[PMID: 15198920]

[3]   Dalrymple U, Mappin B, Gething PW. Malaria mapping: understanding the global endemicity of falciparum and vivax malaria. BMC Med 2015; 13(1): 140.
[http://dx.doi.org/10.1186/s12916-015-0372-x] [PMID: 26071312]

[4]   Khoury MJ, Ioannidis JP. Medicine. Big data meets public health. Science 2003; 339(6123): 275-6.
[PMID: 25430753]

[5]   Collins FS, Varmus H. A new initiative on precision medicine. N Engl J Med 2015; 372(9): 793-5.
[http://dx.doi.org/10.1056/NEJMp1500523] [PMID: 25635347]

[6]   Savitz DA, Goldberg M. Epidemiologic evidence on the health effects of perfluorooctanoic acid (PFOA). Environ Health Perspect 1995; 103 (Suppl. 1): 105-13.

[7]   Islam SMS, Purnat TD, Phuong NTA, Mwingira U, Schacht K, Fröschl G. Non-Communicable Diseases (NCDs) in developing countries: a symposium report. Global Health 2014; 10(1): 81.
[http://dx.doi.org/10.1186/s12992-014-0081-9] [PMID: 25498459]

[8]   Buehler JW, Hopkins RS, Overhage JM, Sosin DM, Tong V. CDC Working Group (2004). Framework for evaluating public health surveillance systems for early detection of outbreaks: recommendations from the CDC Working Group. MMWR Recommendations and reports: Morbidity and mortality weekly report Recommendations and reports. 2004; 53: pp. (RR-5)1-11.

[9]   Heymann D L. Data sharing in public health emergencies: Anthropological and historical reflections on data sharing during the 2014-2016 Ebola epidemic and the 2016 yellow fever epidemic. Data Science and Public Health: Practice and Policy 2015; 49-62.

Real-World Applications and Case Studies in Epidemiology: Bridging Theory and Practice

Abstract: Chapter 7 explores the practical applications of epidemiological principles in various domains, from health policy and evaluation to real-world case studies. Beginning with an introduction to the themes of the chapter, it delves into the implementation of epidemiological concepts in informing health policies and evaluating public health interventions. The chapter also presents compelling case studies that illustrate the application of epidemiological principles in diverse contexts. Furthermore, it offers exercises and questions to engage readers, facilitating active learning and critical thinking in epidemiological practice.

Keywords: Active learning, Case studies, Epidemiological applications, Evaluation, Health policy, Public health interventions.

INTRODUCTION

In our journey through the rich tapestry of epidemiology, we have embarked on an odyssey that has spanned centuries of discovery, traversed the intricacies of models and methods, and reached the forefront of modern science. Now, as we stand on the precipice of a deeper understanding of disease dynamics, we gaze toward the real-world impact of epidemiology—Chapter 7, where the applications and Case Studies of this discipline come to life.

Epidemiology is not an abstract academic pursuit; it is a discipline deeply rooted in the real world, where lives are affected, decisions are made, and public health is advanced. In this chapter, we will voyage through the practical applications of epidemiological knowledge and the enlightening stories of case studies that illuminate its profound impact.

Our journey begins with a voyage into the realm of disease prevention and control. We will explore how epidemiological principles inform public health interventions, from immunization campaigns that have eradicated dead diseases to lifestyle interventions that have curbed the rise of non-communicable conditions. Through engaging narratives, we will witness how epidemiology serves as the guiding light for policymakers and healthcare professionals striving to safeguard the health of populations.

Case studies will provide a window into the remarkable achievements and challenges faced in the field. We will journey to the frontlines of global health, where epidemiologists have battled infectious diseases like Ebola and COVID-19, tracking their spread, formulating containment strategies, and shaping our response to pandemics. These narratives will illustrate the profound impact of epidemiology on the course of history, underscoring its role in shaping the health and well-being of society.

We will also explore the world of environmental epidemiology, where the intersection of human health and the environment is explored. Through case studies, we will unravel the mysteries of how exposure to pollutants, toxins, and climate change can impact human health, illustrating the critical role epidemiology plays in advocating for environmental policies that protect our planet and its inhabitants.

Additionally, we will explore the ethical dimensions of epidemiological research and application, acknowledging the profound responsibility that comes with the pursuit of knowledge that can impact lives. Case studies will illuminate the delicate balance between the quest for scientific truth and the imperative to protect the privacy and well-being of an individual.

As we journey through Chapter 7, remember that epidemiology is not confined to academic halls or research laboratories; it is a dynamic force that shapes public health policies, informs clinical practice, and empowers individuals to make informed decisions about their health. It is the bridge that connects science with action, data with policy, and knowledge with impact.

Welcome to a chapter that showcases the tangible and transformative power of epidemiology, where applications and case studies illustrate its profound reach into the real world. This is where the principles of epidemiology are brought to life, where success stories and challenges inspire us to continue our quest for knowledge and innovation in the relentless pursuit of better health for all.

APPLYING EPIDEMIOLOGICAL PRINCIPLES

Epidemiology plays a pivotal role in shaping *public health interventions* aimed at improving population health [1]. In the context of *public health interventions*, it involves the following:

- **Disease Prevention:** Identifying at-risk populations and developing preventive strategies. For example, implementing vaccination programs to prevent the spread of vaccine-preventable diseases.
- **Health Promotion**: Promoting healthy behaviours and lifestyles through targeted campaigns. This may include anti-smoking initiatives, nutrition education, or physical activity promotion.
- **Health Education:** Providing information and resources to empower individuals and communities to make informed health decisions.
- **Outbreak Response:** Rapidly responding to disease outbreaks by identifying cases, implementing control measures, and preventing further transmission.

Similarly, epidemiological evidence is instrumental in informing health policies at local, national, and global levels [2]. In the context of *health policy development*, the key aspects include:

- **Evidence-Based Policy**: Advocating for policies and regulations grounded in scientific evidence. Epidemiological studies provide the data needed to support policy decisions.
- **Risk Assessment**: Assessing health risks associated with specific behaviours, exposures, or environmental factors. This informs the development of regulations and guidelines.
- **Health Equity**: Identifying health disparities and advocating for policies that reduce inequalities in access to healthcare and health outcomes.

Exercise 1: Designing Local Health Interventions

In this exercise, readers will engage in the process of designing local health interventions based on epidemiological principles:

- **Select a Health Issue**: Choose a prevalent health issue or challenge in your local community or region. This could be a disease, a health behaviour, or a specific population health concern.
- **Review Epidemiological Data:** Examine the available epidemiological data related to the selected health issues. Look for statistics, risk factors, and trends that can inform intervention planning.
- **Identify Target Populations:** Determine the specific populations or groups most affected by the health issue. Consider factors such as age, gender, socioeconomic status, and geographic location.
- **Develop Intervention Strategies:** Based on the epidemiological data and the identified target populations, develop a set of intervention strategies. These could include educational campaigns, community programs, or policy recommendations.

- **Consider Resources:** Assess the resources required for implementing the interventions, including funding, personnel, and infrastructure.
- **Timeline and Evaluation:** Create a timeline for implementing the interventions and outline how you will evaluate their effectiveness. Consider measurable outcomes and evaluation metrics.
- **Engage Stakeholders:** Identify stakeholders and partners who can collaborate on the intervention efforts. This may include local health agencies, community organizations, and healthcare providers.
- **Ethical Considerations:** Reflect on the ethical aspects of the interventions, including issues related to consent, privacy, and equity.

This exercise empowers readers to apply epidemiological principles to real-world scenarios and take an active role in designing and advocating for interventions that address local health challenges. It underscores the practical impact of epidemiology on improving community health and well-being.

EPIDEMIOLOGY IN HEALTH POLICY AND EVALUATION

In the past, epidemiology was not at the fore in shaping health policy formulation, in the development and evaluation of health policies, and in ways that decision-makers would follow to improve the health of the populace. Hitherto, clinicians were guiding policymakers in developing health policies. However, this has changed partly because of globalization and because society is more informed than ever before.

Arguably, 'the role of epidemiology in health policy development and healthcare evaluation' could be considered an area that needs a particular focus. However, because of the importance attached to using findings from epidemiological studies to guide health policy formulation, there is a need for the reader to have an insight into the process of health policy development. The aim of this is to help the reader understand the use of epidemiologic information to guide policy-making and improve the health of the populace [3 - 5].

Health Policy Development

In the epidemiologic context, the outcome of the study of disease distribution and the determinants of health events in a population guides policymakers to develop policies that would prevent and control health problems [3 - 5]. The findings from descriptive studies, which analyse relevant sources of data by person, place, and time, guide public health decision-making bodies. These bodies use the information as a factual framework to help them in policy development, implementation, and evaluation, which culminates in disease prevention and health promotion [3 - 5]. The findings also help these bodies in assessing the health of a population and or communities.

It suffices to say that epidemiologists, using evidence-based strategies, have the responsibility to recommend appropriate interventions and regularly provide guidance and recommendations for use in developing health regulations and healthcare policies. However, in formulating health policies, there is a need to put forward questions that will guide the process; some of these include [3 - 6]:

- How healthy is the population?
- Is there health inequality within the population?
- Do the existing health policies have any impact on the health and quality of life of the people?
- Is there any need for a new health policy?
- What are the existing health problems?
- Are there any available interventions in place to address the health problems?
- Are the current interventions working?
- How can the government make people live healthier?

Again, using baselines and by continuous collection and analysis of the data, epidemiologists help to set health goals for nations, monitor their progress, and help determine how effective and efficient health services are. Similarly, they probe further to know the availability and accessibility of quality healthcare services to every member of the population to know if the health system works at all [3 - 6].

The term policy, which refers to a set of principles that guides decision-making, could broadly be divided into either *systemic or sectoral* policy. Systemic policy, also called macro, looks at the basic characteristics of a society, while *sectoral* policy, also called micro, looks at lower-level decisions [6].

A policy is regarded as a framework that evaluates proposals and measures their progress. Globally, policies are considered critical tools that help governments and organizations to focus and function effectively. Research shows that public health policies target the reduction of social inequalities in health, health promotion, and regulating health-related goods and services [7, 8].

While beyond the scope of this book, it is critical to underscore that policy formulation passes through various stages. There is the 'stage model,' which underscores the usefulness of analytical frameworks in assessing public policies. The 'stage model' simplifies the complex process of public policy development for learners to understand the concept and its applicability. The stages can occur linearly, simultaneously, or in an inverse order and are related to specific activities associated with the policy. While the 'stage model' can vary from five

to seven stages, this book will introduce the reader to Howlett and Ramesh's model, which has five stages [9]:

- **Agenda setting** is all about identifying burning issues of public interest that require the government's attention to propose solutions and to identify groups that would play an active role in addressing the problems.
- **Policy formulation**is the examination of the various policy options for a possible solution. At this stage, the use of the advocacy approach by the coalition groups underscores the problem and possible solution. This stage culminates in setting a policy direction to address the issue.
- **Adoption** is the decision-making stage at the governmental level, and this should align with one or more of the approaches proposed in addressing the problem.
- **Implementation** sets the parameters in place on which the outcome depends. It considers factors that ensure the policy achieves the set objectives. However, the attention is on the technical, administrative, coalition groups, and stakeholders, who must ensure that the policy is implemented to address the problem effectively.
- **Evaluation** is considered the final stage and appraises the formulated policy. The process collects and analyzes information to examine the performance of a program critically. It assesses the level at which the policy is implemented and to know whether the effects have aligned with the set objectives. In addition to engaging government apparatus during this stage, other groups that partake in the process are the consultants or civil society organizations.

However, it is critical to mention that research scientists sometimes experience difficulties in dealing with policymakers during the process of policy formulation. Some of these include lack of political experience, inadequate knowledge of political processes, unrealistic expectations, non-user-friendly platforms to disseminate their scientific results, and the lack of clarity on the implications for costs and impacts of interventions [10].

Healthcare Evaluation

In public health practice, it is through program goals and objectives that criteria and standards are set to evaluate program performance. In evaluating healthcare programs, the information obtained from epidemiological studies plays a critical role. It is critical to mention that a public health program or intervention requires setting strong objectives for use in measuring the output accurately. Thus, the evaluation of a program or intervention can be considered an essential tool for use to analyze whether a program or intervention was able to meet the needs of the end-user. The findings from the evaluation should guide

decision-making and know if there is a need for improvements to program effectiveness [11 - 13].

During program evaluation, there is a need to ask some critical questions that would help to know whether there is a need for improvements, to document the progress, and for the accountability of the policymakers [11 - 13]. This includes the following factors:

- Implementation, to know whether to program is implemented as originally planned.
- Effectiveness, to assess the expected benefits of the healthcare system as measured by improvements in the health of the populace
- Efficiency, as it is related to the appropriate use of resources (human and capital) vis-à-vis the expected outputs or end results
- Cost-effectiveness, as it is related to the benefit of the program vis-à-vis the cost involved.
- Equity, both in terms of accessibility and affordability of healthcare services through fair distribution amongst the citizenry irrespective of social status
- Acceptability, to look at the cultural and social barriers and psychological factors that could hinder people from accessing healthcare services.

The evaluation of the healthcare intervention could either be done at the formative stage (the findings will inform the process) or at the summative stage (to assess the impact). Similarly, depending on the healthcare program, the evaluation can either be prospective or retrospective. It is critical to emphasize that the process of evaluating a healthcare system would require setting objectives [11 - 13]. This includes the use of SMART objectives:

S - specific (to look at effectiveness, efficiency, equity, acceptability)

M - measurable

A - achievable

R - realistic (within available resources)

T – time-bound (within a set timeline)

Although there are different stages for program evaluation, there are four stages that are commonly used: planning, implementation, completion, and reporting.

- *Planning* requires prioritizing short and long-term goals, identifying the target audience, determining the methods of data collection, and assessing the feasibility.
- *Implementation*, at this stage, might focus on the formative and process evaluation strategies.
- *Completion* depends on the evaluation plan and could come either midway or at the end of the program. Importantly, the focus would be to examine the long-term outcomes and impacts and to summarize the overall performance of the program.
- *Reporting* is how to report and effectively communicate the findings of the project. The emphasis here is to select the right target audiences and the medium to disseminate the findings.

Thus, in healthcare evaluation, the reader should be able to distinguish between the principles of research and that of program evaluation, as highlighted in Table **1** [12, 13].

Table 1. Distinguishing principles of research and evaluation [12, 13].

Concept	Research Principles	Program Evaluation Principles
Planning	**Scientific method**	**Framework for program evaluation**
-	1. State hypothesis.	1. Engage stakeholders.
-	2. Collect data.	2. Describe the program.
-	3. Analyze data.	3. Focus evaluation design.
-	4. Draw conclusions.	4. Gather credible evidence.
-	-	5. Justify conclusions.
-	-	6. Ensure use and share the lessons learned.
Decision Making	**Investigator-controlled**	**Stakeholder-controlled**
-	1. Authoritative.	1. Collaborative.
Standards	**Validity**	**Repeatability program evaluation standards**
-	1. Internal (accuracy, precision).	1. Utility.
-	2. External (generalizability).	2. Feasibility.
-	-	3. Propriety.
-	-	4. Accuracy
Questions	**Facts**	**Values**
-	1. Descriptions	1. Merit (*i.e.*, quality).
-	2. Associations	2. Worth (*i.e.*, value).
-	3. Effects.	3. Significance (*i.e.*, importance).

(Table 1) cont.....

Concept	Research Principles	Program Evaluation Principles
Design	**Isolate changes and control circumstances**	**Incorporate changes and account for circumstances**
-	1. Narrow experimental influences.	1. Expand to see all domains of influence.
-	2. Ensure stability over time.	2. Encourage flexibility and improvement.
-	3. Minimize context dependence.	3. Maximize context sensitivity.
-	4. Treat contextual factors as confounding (*e.g.*, randomization, adjustment, statistical control).	4. Treat contextual factors as essential information (*e.g.*, system diagrams, logic models, hierarchical or ecological modeling).
-	5. Understand that comparison groups are a necessity	5. Understand that comparisons between groups are optional (and sometimes harmful).
Data Collection	**Sources**	**Sources**
-	1. Limited number (accuracy preferred).	1. Multiple (triangulation preferred).
-	2. Sampling strategies are critical.	2. Sampling strategies are critical.
-	3. Concern for protecting human subjects.	3. Concern for protecting human subjects, organizations, and communities.
-	**Indicators/Measures**	**Indicators/Measures**
-	1. Quantitative.	1. Mixed methods (qualitative, quantitative, and integrated).
-	2. Qualitative.	-
Analysis and Synthesis	**Timing**	**Timing**
-	One time (at the end).	Ongoing (formative and summative).
-	**Scope**	**Scope**
-	Focus on specific variables.	Integrate all data.
Judgements	**Implicit**	**Explicit**
-	Attempt to remain value-free.	1. Examine agreement on values.
-	-	2. State precisely whose values are used.
Conclusions	**Attribution**	**Attribution and contribution**
-	1. Establish the time sequence.	1. Establish the time sequence.
-	2. Demonstrate plausible mechanisms.	2. Demonstrate plausible mechanisms.
-	3. Control for confounding.	3. Account for alternative explanations.
-	4. Replicate findings.	-
-	-	**Feedback to stakeholders**
-	-	1. Focus on intended use by intended users.
-	-	2. Build capacity.
Uses	**Disseminate to interested audiences**	**Disseminate to interested audiences**

(Table 1) cont.....

Concept	Research Principles	Program Evaluation Principles
-	Content and format vary to maximize comprehension.	1. Content and format vary to maximize comprehension.
-	-	2. Emphasis on full disclosure
-	-	3. Requirements for balanced assessment

CASE STUDIES IN EPIDEMIOLOGICAL PRACTICE

Real-World Applications

In this section, we delve into real-world case studies that exemplify the practical applications of epidemiological principles. These case studies encompass a wide range of health issues and scenarios, providing insights into how epidemiology informs decision-making and intervention strategies [14].

- **Infectious Disease Outbreak Response**: Explore case studies of rapid response to infectious disease outbreaks, such as Zika virus, Ebola, or foodborne illness outbreaks. Learn how epidemiologists identify the source and transmission dynamics and implement control measures.
- **Chronic Disease Prevention:** Examine examples of successful interventions aimed at reducing the prevalence of chronic diseases like heart disease, diabetes, and cancer. Discover how epidemiological data informs lifestyle interventions and healthcare policies.
- **Environmental Health Challenges:** Investigate cases related to environmental health, including air pollution, water contamination, and occupational hazards. Understand how epidemiology plays a role in assessing exposure risks and advocating for environmental regulation.

Problem-Solving in Epidemiology

Epidemiologists are often confronted with complex health challenges that require innovative problem-solving [15]. This section highlights how epidemiology tackles such challenges:

- **Emergency Preparedness and Response**: Learn about epidemiological strategies for disaster preparedness and response. Explore how epidemiologists coordinate with emergency agencies to protect public health during natural disasters or bioterrorism events.
- **Vaccine Development and Immunization Programs:** Delve into the epidemiological research behind vaccine development and immunization programs. Understand how epidemiologists assess vaccine safety and effectiveness.

- **Global Health Equity:** Investigate case studies related to global health disparities and inequalities. Discover how epidemiological research informs initiatives aimed at reducing health inequities worldwide.

Exercise 2: Solving Local Health Challenges Through Epidemiology

In this exercise, readers will actively engage in problem-solving by applying epidemiological approaches to address local health challenges:

- **Identify a Local Health Challenge:** Choose a specific health challenge or issue in your local community or region that you are passionate about addressing. It could be related to a disease, a health behavior, or a healthcare system challenge.
- **Analyze Epidemiological Data:** Collect and analyze relevant epidemiological data related to the chosen health challenge. Utilize available statistics, research studies, or local health department reports.
- **Identify Key Determinants:** Determine the key determinants or factors contributing to the health challenge. Consider both proximal and distal causes, as well as social determinants of health.
- **Propose Interventions**: Develop a set of evidence-based interventions to address the identified determinants. These interventions should be actionable and have the potential to bring about positive change.
- **Consider Ethical and Equity Considerations:** Reflect on ethical considerations related to your proposed intervention, including issues of consent, privacy, and fairness. Ensure that your interventions prioritize health equity.
- **Engage Stakeholders:** Identify stakeholders and partners who can collaborate on implementing your proposed interventions. Consider how to involve the affected community in the decision-making process.
- **Create an Implementation Plan:** Outline a comprehensive plan for implementing your proposed interventions, including timelines, resource requirements, and evaluation metrics.

This exercise empowers readers to take on the role of epidemiologists and actively contribute to solving local health challenges. It underscores the practical and problem-solving aspect of epidemiology, emphasizing its potential to drive positive change and improve community health outcomes.

EXERCISES AND QUESTIONS FOR READERS

Applying Knowledge to Local and Current Health Issues

In this section, we provide exercises and questions designed to encourage readers to actively apply the knowledge they have gained throughout the book to address local and current health challenges. These exercises aim to empower readers to become effective epidemiological problem solvers in their communities.

Exercise 3: Applying Epidemiological Principles to Local Health Challenges

- **Select a Local Health Challenge:** Choose a specific health issue or challenge in your local community that requires attention. This could be an infectious disease outbreak, a chronic health problem, or a health behavior concern.
- **Epidemiological Assessment**: Conduct an epidemiological assessment of the selected health challenge. Gather relevant data, statistics, and information to understand the scope and determinants of the problem.
- **Identify Key Determinants:** Determine the key determinants contributing to the health challenge. Consider factors, such as demographics, socioeconomic status, environmental influences, and lifestyle behaviors.
- **Propose Evidence-Based Interventions**: Based on your epidemiological assessment, we propose evidence-based interventions to address the identified determinants. These interventions should be feasible and tailored to the local context.
- **Ethical Considerations:** Discuss the ethical considerations associated with your proposed interventions. Consider issues related to informed consent, privacy, and justice.
- **Community Engagement:** Explore strategies for engaging the affected community in the decision-making process and implementation of interventions. How can community input and involvement be maximized?
- **Implementation Plan:** Create a detailed plan for implementing your proposed interventions. Outline the steps, resources, and timelines required for each intervention.

Questions for Reflection and Discussion

1. How does epidemiology contribute to evidence-based decision-making in public health and healthcare policy? Provide examples from your region or country.

2. What are the primary challenges in applying epidemiological principles to address health disparities and promote health equity in your community?

3. Consider a recent health issue or outbreak in your area. How could the principles of epidemiology have been applied to better understand and control the situation?

4. Discuss the role of community engagement in epidemiological research and public health interventions. How can communities be actively involved in the research process and decision-making?

5. Reflect on the ethical considerations that arise in epidemiological research and practice. What ethical principles should guide epidemiologists in their work?

6. Explore the concept of One Health, which emphasizes the interconnectedness of human, animal, and environmental health. How can One Health approach benefit public health efforts in your region?

These exercises and questions encourage readers to think critically about the application of epidemiological principles to address local health challenges. They prompt readers to consider the ethical, practical, and community-oriented aspects of epidemiological practice and research. By engaging with these exercises and questions, readers can deepen their understanding and develop practical skills in epidemiology that are directly applicable to their communities and regions.

CONCLUSION

In conclusion, Chapter 7 has provided a comprehensive exploration of the practical applications of epidemiological principles, encompassing health policy evaluation and real-world case studies. By examining the role of epidemiology in informing public health practice and policy, readers have gained valuable insights into the diverse applications of epidemiological research and practice. Moreover, the chapter underscores the importance of active learning and critical thinking in epidemiological practice, offering exercises and questions to engage readers in further exploration of key concepts. As readers continue to engage with the material presented in the chapter, they will deepen their understanding of epidemiological applications and their impact on improving population health outcomes.

REFERENCES

[1]   Brownson RC, Baker EA, Leet TL, Gillespie KN. Evidence-Based Public Health. 3rd ed., Oxford University Press 2016.

[2]   Buse K, Mays N, Walt G. Making Health Policy. McGraw-Hill Education 2012.

[3]   Bonita R, Beaglehole R, Kjellström T. Basic epidemiology. 2nd ed., World Health Organ 2006.

[4]   An Introduction to Applied Epidemiology and Biostatistics. Principles of Epidemiology in Public Health Practice. 3rd ed. Atlanta, GA: Centers for Disease Control and Prevention 2012; p. 30333.

[5]   Available   from: https://www.who.int/emergencies/diseases/novel-coronavirus-2019/events-as--hey-happen

[6]   Spasoff RA. 1999. Epidemiologic methods for health policy. Oxford University Press, Inc.

[7]   Barata RB. Epidemiology and public policies. Rev. bras. epidemiol. 2013; 16(1). ISSN 1415-790X.

[http://dx.doi.org/10.1590/S1415-790X2013000100001]

[8]   Petticrew M, Whitehead M, Macintyre SJ, Graham H, Egan M. Evidence for public health policy on inequalities: 1: The reality according to policymakers. J Epidemiol Community Health 2004; 58(10): 811-6.
[http://dx.doi.org/10.1136/jech.2003.015289] [PMID: 15365104]

[9]   Benoit F. Public Policy Models and Their Usefulness in Public Health: The Stages Model. Montréal, Québec: National Collaborating Centre for Healthy Public Policy 2013.

[10]   Martin R, Conseil A, Longstaff A, *et al.* Pandemic influenza control in Europe and the constraints resulting from incoherent public health laws. BMC Public Health 2010; 10(1): 532.
[http://dx.doi.org/10.1186/1471-2458-10-532] [PMID: 20815888]

[11]   Patton MQ. Qualitative Research Evaluation Methods. Thousand Oaks, CA: Sage Publishers 1987.

[12]   Green LW, George MA, Daniel M, *et al.* Study of participatory research in health promotion: Review and recommendations for the development of participatory research in health promotion in Canada. Ottawa, Canada: Royal Society of Canada 1995.

[13]   Introduction to program evaluation for public health programs: A self-study guide US Department of Health and Human Services. Atlanta, GA: Centers for Disease Control and Prevention 2011.

[14]   Koopman JS, Lynch JW. Individual causal models and population system models in epidemiology. Am J Public Health 1999; 89(8): 1170-4.
[http://dx.doi.org/10.2105/AJPH.89.8.1170] [PMID: 10432901]

[15]   Rothman KJ, Greenland S, Lash TL. Modern Epidemiology. 3rd ed., Lippincott Williams & Wilkins 2008.

CHAPTER 8

Navigating the Future: Innovations, Ethical Dilemmas, and the Path Forward in Epidemiology

Abstract: Chapter 8 navigates the evolving landscape of epidemiology, exploring innovations, ethical considerations, and prospects for shaping the future of this field. Beginning with an introduction to the themes of the chapter, it delves into recent innovations in epidemiological methods, offering insights into emerging approaches and technologies. The chapter also addresses the ethical considerations inherent in epidemiological research, highlighting the importance of ethical practice in safeguarding participant welfare and research integrity. Furthermore, it discusses strategies for shaping the future of epidemiology, emphasizing the need for interdisciplinary collaboration and proactive engagement with emerging challenges.

Keywords: Challenges, Epidemiology, Ethical Considerations, Future directions, Innovations, Interdisciplinary Collaboration, Public Health, Research Integrity.

INTRODUCTION

As we approach the culmination of our expedition through the vast landscape of epidemiology, we stand at a crossroads between the known and the unknown, the present and the future. Chapter 8 beckons us to peer into the horizon, where the contours of epidemiology are ever-shifting, and the challenges we face are as dynamic as the world we inhabit. Welcome to the realm of "Future Directions and Challenges."

Epidemiology, like the diseases it studies, is in a state of constant evolution. It is a discipline shaped not only by the past but also by the aspirations and innovations of the future. In this chapter, we embark on a forward-looking journey, exploring the emerging trends, the uncharted territories, and the enduring challenges that will define the trajectory of epidemiology in the years to come.

Our journey begins by peering into the crystal ball of epidemiological innovation. We will delve into the potential of genomics, precision medicine, and digital health technologies to revolutionize our understanding of diseases and tailor interventions to individual needs. From the promise of personalized risk assessment to the possibility of predicting disease outbreaks with unprecedented accuracy, the future of epidemiology is awash with exciting possibilities.

We will also explore the expanding role of interdisciplinary collaboration in epidemiology. In an era where complex health challenges demand holistic solutions, we will witness how partnerships between epidemiologists, data scientists, social scientists, and policymakers foster a convergence of knowledge that holds the key to solving some of our most pressing health problems.

However, with innovation comes responsibility. We will confront the ethical and societal challenges as epidemiology navigates the uncharted waters of genetic information, big data, and artificial intelligence. Questions of privacy, equity, and transparency will arise, and we must navigate them with wisdom and foresight.

Epidemiology does not exist in isolation; it is intrinsically intertwined with the societal forces that shape our health. We will explore how epidemiology can be a catalyst for addressing social determinants of health, advocating for health equity, and tackling emerging global health threats, from climate change to antimicrobial resistance.

As we peer into the future, we must also acknowledge the persistent challenges that epidemiology faces. The battle against infectious diseases is ongoing, and new threats will inevitably emerge. Chronic diseases continue to burden populations worldwide, demanding innovative approaches to prevention and management. The ever-expanding realm of environmental health poses new questions about the intersection of the well-being of our planet and human health.

In Chapter 8, we confront the reality that pursuing epidemiological knowledge is an unending journey. The challenges may evolve, but so does our determination to meet them with courage and intellect. We must equip the next generation of epidemiologists with the tools and skills to navigate this complex terrain and steer the course toward a healthier world.

Welcome to a chapter that serves as both a compass and a call to action for the future of epidemiology. "Future Directions and Challenges" invites us to embrace uncertainty with curiosity, address challenges with resilience, and envision a world where epidemiology continues to illuminate the path toward better health and well-being for all.

INNOVATIONS IN EPIDEMIOLOGICAL METHODS

Epidemiology stands as a cornerstone discipline in the ever-evolving landscape of public health and disease prevention. Its role in understanding the spread of diseases, identifying risk factors, and guiding public health interventions has been pivotal throughout history. However, as the challenges of the modern world become increasingly complex and interconnected, the field of epidemiology has to adapt and innovate to keep pace with the evolving landscape of health threats [1, 2].

In this chapter, we embark on a journey through cutting-edge methodologies, techniques, and technologies reshaping how we approach epidemiology. These innovations enhance our ability to track and control diseases and offer fresh insights into the intricate web of factors influencing our health [1, 2].

Epidemiologists are no longer confined to traditional data collection and analysis techniques. Instead, they are harnessing the power of big data, artificial intelligence, advanced statistical models, and interdisciplinary collaboration to uncover patterns and trends that were once hidden from view. This chapter explores how these innovations revolutionise our understanding of diseases and transform how we design and implement public health strategies [1, 2].

From the use of genomic epidemiology to trace the origins of infectious outbreaks to the application of machine learning algorithms to predict disease outbreaks, this chapter provides a comprehensive overview of the exciting developments shaping the future of epidemiology. We also examine the ethical considerations and challenges of these innovations, ensuring that we balance scientific progress and responsible data use.

As the world continues to evolve, so do the methods and tools available to epidemiologists. These innovations are enabling us to tackle complex health challenges more effectively than ever before.

Big Data, Artificial Intelligence, and Machine Learning

In an era of information abundance and technological leaps, the convergence of Big Data, Artificial Intelligence (AI), and Machine Learning (ML) represents a transformative force with far-reaching implications. As we stand on the precipice of the Fourth Industrial Revolution, these three pillars of innovation have become the cornerstones of progress, shaping industries, redefining research, and revolutionising our understanding of the world [1].

This section delves deep into the exciting realm of "Big Data, Artificial Intelligence, and Machine Learning." Here, we embark on a journey through the digital landscape where data, algorithms, and human ingenuity converge to unlock the vast potential of these technologies [1].

Big Data has opened new vistas of discovery in healthcare and finance. Coupled with AI and ML, this data-driven revolution has empowered us to unravel complex patterns, make predictions with unprecedented accuracy, and automate tasks once thought to be the exclusive domain of human intelligence [1].

However, with great power comes great responsibility. As we harness the capabilities of Big Data, AI, and ML, we must also grapple with ethical and societal implications. It is essential to emphasise the importance of balancing innovation and responsible stewardship [1].

- *Big Data:* The proliferation of digital information has given rise to big data, which encompasses vast datasets that can be collected, stored, and analyzed. In epidemiology, big data can include electronic health records, social media data, and genomic information. These data sources provide unprecedented insights into health trends and patterns.
- *Artificial Intelligence (AI):* AI refers to the development of computer systems that can perform tasks that typically require human intelligence, such as learning from data, reasoning, and problem-solving. In epidemiology, AI is being used to analyze large datasets quickly and accurately, identify disease outbreaks in real time, and predict disease trends.
- *Machine Learning (ML):* ML is a subset of AI that focuses on the development of algorithms that enable computers to learn from and make predictions or decisions based on data. In epidemiology, ML algorithms are used to identify patterns in health data, detect early warning signs of disease outbreaks, and personalize treatment plans for individuals.

Future Trends in Epidemiology

Epidemiology, the science of understanding the patterns and determinants of health and disease in populations, has been at the forefront of public health for centuries. Its invaluable role in identifying and combating infectious diseases, chronic conditions, and emerging health threats has saved countless lives and improved the well-being of communities worldwide [2]. As we enter an era of unprecedented change and complexity, epidemiology stands poised to evolve and adapt to the unique challenges of the future.

This section introduces the reader to the dynamics and ever-evolving landscape of "Future Trends in Epidemiology." Here, we embark on a journey through the exciting possibilities and transformative forces that promise to shape the discipline in the coming years. The practice of epidemiology is no longer confined to traditional methods of data collection and analysis. In this chapter, we venture into precision epidemiology, genomics, digital health, and global interconnectedness [2].

1. *Precision Epidemiology:* Precision epidemiology is a relatively new approach to public health that seeks to tailor interventions and health strategies to the individual characteristics of specific populations or even individual patients. This approach recognizes that not all individuals are affected by disease or respond to treatment similarly. It considers genetics, lifestyle, environment, and socio-economic status to provide more targeted and personalized healthcare solutions.

- *Genetic Variation:* Precision epidemiology often incorporates genetic information to identify genetic predispositions to certain diseases. Understanding the genetic makeup of an an individual can help predict disease risk and guide personalized prevention and treatment strategies.
- *Lifestyle Factors*: Precision epidemiology considers lifestyle factors, such as diet, physical activity, and habits like smoking or alcohol consumption. Tailoring recommendations to the lifestyle of an individual can increase the likelihood of behaviour change.
- *Environmental Exposures:* This approach also accounts for environmental factors, such as air and water quality, exposure to toxins, and geographical location, which can impact health outcomes. Precision epidemiology may involve mapping environmental exposures to identify high-risk areas.

2. *Genomics:* Genomics studies the complete set of genes (its genome) of an organism and their interactions. In epidemiology, genomics has become increasingly crucial for understanding the genetic underpinnings of diseases and how they spread within populations.

- *Disease Susceptibility:* Genomics helps identify genetic variations associated with disease susceptibility. By studying the genetic profiles of individuals and populations, researchers can pinpoint genetic markers that increase or decrease the risk of certain diseases.
- *Pharmacogenomics:* This subfield focuses on how the genetic makeup of an individual influences their medication response. It allows for the development of personalized medicine by tailoring drug treatments to their genetic profile.
- *Genomic Epidemiology*: Genomic epidemiology combines genomic data with traditional epidemiological methods to trace the origins of diseases, especially infectious ones. It aids in understanding how pathogens evolve and spread in populations.

3. *Digital Health:* Digital health refers to using digital technologies, including mobile apps, wearables, telemedicine, electronic health records, and data analytics, to improve healthcare delivery, monitoring, and patient outcomes.

- ***Wearable Devices***: These devices, such as smartwatches and fitness trackers, collect real-time health data like heart rate, activity levels, and sleep patterns. This data can be used for disease monitoring, early detection, and promoting healthy behaviours.
- ***Telemedicine***: Digital health enables remote healthcare consultations, making it easier for individuals to access medical advice and treatment. It is especially valuable in rural or underserved areas.
- ***Electronic Health Records (EHRs)***:EHRs store the medical information of patients electronically, facilitating data sharing among healthcare providers and improving patient care coordination.
- ***Data Analytics***: Advanced analytics and machine learning are used to process and analyze vast amounts of health data, offering insights for disease surveillance, treatment recommendations, and health management.

4. *Global Interconnectedness:* Global interconnectedness refers to the increasing interdependence of countries and regions, including trade, travel, information exchange, and disease spread. It profoundly affects epidemiology in the following ways:

- ***Disease Transmission***: Diseases can spread rapidly across borders due to increased travel and trade. Epidemiologists must collaborate internationally to monitor and control outbreaks effectively.
- ***Data Sharing***: Global interconnectedness requires better sharing of epidemiological data and information between countries to promptly respond to emerging health threats.
- ***One Health Approach:*** This approach recognizes the interconnectedness of human, animal, and environmental health. It is vital for addressing zoonotic diseases that can jump from animals to humans.
- ***Global Health Governance***: To manage global health challenges, organizations like the World Health Organization (WHO) are crucial in coordinating responses and setting international health standards.

These concepts collectively represent the evolving landscape of epidemiology, where precision, genetics, digital tools, and global cooperation redefine how we understand, prevent, and respond to health challenges. They empower epidemiologists to tailor interventions, harness genetic insights, leverage technology, and work collaboratively globally to protect and improve public health.

Exercise 1: Exploring Innovations in Epidemiology

To better understand these innovations, consider the following questions and exercises:

- **Big Data Exploration:** Research and identify examples of how big data has been used in epidemiology to address health challenges. How has it improved our understanding of disease trends?
- **AI and ML in Health:** Explore how artificial intelligence and machine learning are being applied in healthcare and epidemiology. Are there specific applications that stand out in your region or community?
- **Future Trends Discussion:** Engage in discussions or group activities to brainstorm how precision epidemiology, the one health approach, and global health security could be applied to address local health issues or challenges.
- **Personal Reflection:** Reflect on how these innovations might impact your future work or research in epidemiology. What opportunities and challenges do they present?

By exploring these innovations and considering their implications, readers can gain a deeper understanding of the rapidly evolving field of epidemiology and its potential to shape the future of public health.

ETHICAL CONSIDERATIONS IN EPIDEMIOLOGICAL RESEARCH

Epidemiological research involves collecting, analyzing, and interpreting data related to health and diseases. It is imperative that this research is conducted with the highest ethical standards to protect the rights, privacy, and well-being of study participants and communities [3, 4]. This section explores critical ethical considerations in epidemiological research.

Privacy and Data Security

1. *Data Privacy:* Epidemiological research often deals with sensitive health information about individuals and populations. Researchers must prioritize data privacy by obtaining informed consent from participants and ensuring that their data are anonymized or de-identified to prevent any possibility of identifying individuals.

2. *Data Security:* With the increasing reliance on electronic health records and digital data collection methods, data security is paramount. Researchers must implement robust data security measures to protect data against breaches, unauthorized access, and cyber threats.

Ethical Use of Emerging Technologies

1. *Emerging Technologies:* As epidemiology embraces innovations like big data analytics, artificial intelligence, and genomics, researchers encounter new ethical challenges. These technologies offer unprecedented opportunities for insight but also pose risks such as bias, discrimination, and infringement on individual privacy.

2. *Informed Consent:* In the context of emerging technologies, ensuring that study participants fully understand the implications of data collection, analysis, and potential consequences is crucial. Researchers must uphold the principles of informed consent and transparency.

Exercise 2: Addressing Ethical Challenges in Research

To deepen understanding and engagement with ethical considerations, readers can participate in exercises and discussions:

- **Privacy Assessment:** Reflect on the state of data privacy and security in your region or community. Are there existing laws or regulations that protect the health data of individuals? Identify any gaps or areas that require improvement.
- **Case Studies:** Analyze real-world examples of ethical dilemmas in epidemiological research involving emerging technologies. Discuss how these challenges were addressed or how they could have been handled more ethically.
- **Ethical Guidelines:** Explore and discuss ethical guidelines and principles for epidemiological research provided by international organizations and regulatory bodies. Consider how these guidelines can be practically applied in local research contexts.

By actively engaging in discussions and exercises related to ethical considerations, readers can develop a deeper appreciation for the ethical complexities of epidemiological research and contribute to the responsible conduct of research in their local contexts.

SHAPING THE FUTURE OF EPIDEMIOLOGY

The field of epidemiology is continuously evolving, driven by emerging health challenges, technological advancements, and changing societal needs [5, 6]. This section focuses on how epidemiologists can actively shape the future of the discipline and make a tangible impact on public health.

Advocacy and Policymaking

1. Epidemiologists as Advocates: Epidemiologists are uniquely positioned to advocate for evidence-based policies and interventions. They can bridge the gap between research and policymaking by translating complex findings into actionable recommendations for decision-makers.

2. Community Engagement: Effective advocacy often requires engaging with the communities affected by health issues. Epidemiologists can facilitate community involvement in policymaking processes, ensuring that policies are culturally sensitive and meet the specific needs of the population.

Interdisciplinary Collaboration

1. The Power of Collaboration: Many health challenges today are multifaceted, requiring expertise from various disciplines. Epidemiologists can collaborate with experts in fields such as sociology, economics, environmental science, and genetics to gain a holistic understanding of complex health issues.

2. Translational Research: Interdisciplinary collaboration can lead to translational research, where scientific discoveries are translated into practical applications. Epidemiologists can work with clinicians, researchers, and policymakers to bridge the gap between laboratory findings and real-world health interventions.

Exercise 3: Advocating for Health Policy Change in Your Region

To empower readers to take an active role in shaping the future of epidemiology and public health in their communities, this exercise encourages advocacy and engagement:

- **Identify Local Health Issues:** Research and identify pressing health issues in your region or community. Consider factors like disease prevalence, social determinants of health, and healthcare access.
- **Policy Analysis:** Examine existing health policies related to the identified issues. Assess their effectiveness, relevance, and alignment with current research findings.
- **Advocacy Plan:** Develop an advocacy plan outlining specific steps to advocate for policy changes. This may involve engaging with local policymakers, conducting awareness campaigns, or collaborating with community organizations.
- **Community Engagement:** Engage with community members, healthcare professionals, and relevant stakeholders to gather support for your advocacy

efforts. Consider organizing community meetings, workshops, or online forums to raise awareness and build a coalition for change.

• **Advocacy Actions:** Implement your advocacy plan, taking actions, such as meeting with policymakers, presenting research findings, or organizing public events. Monitor progress and adapt your approach as needed.

By participating in Exercise 3, readers can actively contribute to improving public health policies and promoting evidence-based decision-making in their region, thereby shaping the future of epidemiology and healthcare.

CONCLUSION

In conclusion, Chapter 8 has offered a comprehensive exploration of future directions and challenges in epidemiology, encompassing innovations, ethical considerations, and strategies for shaping the trajectory of this field. By examining recent innovations and ethical considerations, readers have gained valuable insights into the evolving landscape of epidemiological research and practice. Moreover, the chapter underscores the importance of interdisciplinary collaboration and proactive engagement in addressing emerging challenges and shaping the future of epidemiology. As readers continue to engage with the material presented in the chapter, they will further deepen their understanding of the dynamic nature of this field and its pivotal role in advancing public health.

REFERENCES

[1]   Obermeyer Z, Emanuel EJ. Predicting the Future — Big Data, Machine Learning, and Clinical Medicine. N Engl J Med 2016; 375(13): 1216-9.
[http://dx.doi.org/10.1056/NEJMp1606181] [PMID: 27682033]

[2]   Rocklöv J, Sjödin H. High population densities catalyse the spread of COVID-19. J Travel Med 2020; 27(3): taaa038.
[http://dx.doi.org/10.1093/jtm/taaa038] [PMID: 32227186]

[3]   Gostin LO, Hodge JG Jr. US emergency legal responses to novel coronavirus: Balancing public health and civil liberties. JAMA 2020; 323(12): 1131-2.
[http://dx.doi.org/10.1001/jama.2020.2025] [PMID: 32207808]

[4]   Saldaña J. Ethical challenges of digital health technologies: Lessons learned from a qualitative study of older adults. J Ethics Law Aging 2020; 26(2): 143-62.

[5]   Brownson RC, Fielding JE, Green LW. Building capacity for evidence-based public health: Reconciling the pulls of practice and the push of research. Annu Rev Public Health 2024; 39(1): 27-53.
[http://dx.doi.org/10.1146/annurev-publhealth-040617-014746] [PMID: 29166243]

[6]   Stokols D, Hall KL, Taylor BK, Moser RP. The science of team science: overview of the field and introduction to the supplement. Am J Prev Med 2008; 35(2) (Suppl.): S77-89.
[http://dx.doi.org/10.1016/j.amepre.2008.05.002] [PMID: 18619407]

Epidemiology in Local Context

Abstract: Chapter 9 explores the application of epidemiological principles within specific regional and community settings. Beginning with an introduction to the themes of the chapter, it delves into the adaptation of epidemiological methods to address the unique challenges and characteristics of different regions. The chapter emphasizes the importance of community engagement in epidemiological practice, highlighting strategies for fostering collaboration and building trust within local populations. Through compelling case studies, readers gain insights into the practical application of epidemiological principles in addressing health disparities and promoting community well-being at the grassroots level.

Keywords: Adaptation, Community engagement, Case studies, Epidemiology, Health disparities, Local context, Public health, Regional challenges.

INTRODUCTION

Epidemiology, the science of understanding and managing the health of populations, is often seen as a global endeavour. We explore pandemics that span continents, study data from nations far and wide, and seek universal truths about the spread of diseases. Nevertheless, at the heart of this expansive field lies a crucial principle—that the health of individuals and communities is profoundly influenced by the unique characteristics of their local context.

Chapter 9 beckons us to focus on scrutinizing the intricate dynamics of epidemiology within the confines of local communities. Welcome to "Epidemiology in Local Context," where we illuminate the microcosm within the macrocosm, where the science of epidemiology finds its most tangible expression in the neighbourhoods, towns, and regions where people live, work, and thrive.

Local context matters. It shapes the fabric of our daily lives, influencing our health behaviours, access to healthcare, and exposure to risks. Whether it is the air we breathe, the water we drink, or the socioeconomic conditions we experience, the health of a community reflects its local context. In this chapter, we explore how epidemiology becomes a powerful tool for deciphering and addressing the intricacies of these local contexts.

We start by recognizing that the health challenges different communities face are as diverse as the landscapes they inhabit. From urban centres grappling with the health implications of rapid urbanization to rural communities contending with limited access to healthcare, every locale presents a unique set of epidemiological puzzles. We will journey through case studies that shed light on the localized epidemics, clusters, and disparities that require tailored interventions.

Local context extends beyond the physical environment. Cultural beliefs, social norms, and community structures play a pivotal role in shaping health outcomes. We will explore how epidemiologists work in close partnership with local communities, engaging in culturally sensitive research and co-design interventions that respect and honour the diverse values and traditions that define the fabric of our society.

Public health is not a one-size-fits-all discipline. The solutions that work in one community may not be effective in another. We will witness how epidemiologists adapt their methods and strategies to address the specific needs and challenges of local contexts, promoting health equity and ensuring that no community is left behind.

In this chapter, we will also confront the ethical considerations when conducting research in local contexts, acknowledging the importance of community engagement, informed consent, and responsible use of data. We will see how ethical principles are not just theoretical concepts but practical guidelines that guide the work of epidemiologists on the ground.

"Epidemiology in Local Context" is a reminder that while our gaze may often be drawn to the global stage, it is at the local level where the impact of epidemiology is most keenly observed. This chapter invites us to appreciate the diversity of challenges and opportunities within our communities and recognize the critical role that local epidemiology plays in safeguarding and improving the health of those we know and love.

Welcome to a chapter that celebrates the power of epidemiology to make a tangible difference in the lives of individuals and communities, where the pursuit of health begins in our neighbourhoods and where the science of epidemiology finds its most meaningful expression in the local context.

ADAPTING EPIDEMIOLOGICAL METHODS TO YOUR REGION

Epidemiology is a versatile field, and its methods can be adapted to suit the unique characteristics and challenges of different regions and populations [1, 2].

This section explores the importance of tailoring epidemiological approaches to the local context.

Cultural and Social Considerations

1. Understanding Cultural Sensitivity: Epidemiologists must recognize the cultural diversity of the populations they work with. Cultural beliefs, practices, and norms can significantly impact health behaviors and outcomes. It is essential to approach research and interventions with cultural sensitivity to build trust and relevance within communities.

2. Community Engagement: Building strong relationships with local communities is crucial. Epidemiologists should collaborate with community leaders, organizations, and individuals to understand cultural nuances, gain insights into health-related behaviors, and co-design interventions that resonate with the values of the community.

Local Epidemiological Challenges

1. Identifying Regional Health Priorities: Different regions face distinct health challenges. Epidemiologists should prioritize research and interventions that address the most pressing health issues in their area. This might involve conducting a needs assessment to identify local priorities.

2. Resource Constraints: Resource limitations can pose challenges to epidemiological research and public health initiatives. Understanding the available resources and seeking innovative and cost-effective solutions are essential for making a meaningful impact in resource-constrained settings.

Exercise 1: Tailoring Epidemiological Approaches to Your Local Context

This exercise encourages readers to apply the principles discussed in this chapter to adapt epidemiological methods to their specific local context:

- **Identify Local Health Issues**: Choose a specific health issue or challenge that is prevalent in your region or community. Consider factors such as disease prevalence, social determinants of health, and local priorities.
- **Cultural Assessment:** Conduct a cultural assessment to understand the cultural beliefs, practices, and norms that may influence health-related behaviors and attitudes in your community. Engage with community members and leaders to gain insight.

- **Local Challenges**: Identify any unique challenges or constraints that may affect epidemiological research or public health interventions in your region. These could include resource limitations, geographic barriers, or social disparities.
- **Tailored Approach:** Develop a tailored approach to address the identified health issue in your local context. Consider how cultural and social considerations can be integrated into research design, data collection, and intervention strategies.
- **Community Engagement:** Outline plan for engaging with the local community throughout the epidemiological process. Describe how you will build trust, involve community members in decision-making, and ensure that interventions are culturally relevant.
- **Implementation:** Put your tailored approach into action. Conduct research, implement interventions, or advocate for policy changes based on your adapted epidemiological methods.

By completing Exercise 1, readers can gain practical experience in adapting epidemiological methods to their specific region or community, ultimately enhancing the effectiveness and relevance of public health efforts in their local context.

COMMUNITY ENGAGEMENT AND EPIDEMIOLOGICAL PRACTICE

Community engagement is a cornerstone of effective epidemiological practice. This section delves into the importance of building partnerships with local communities and conducting community-based research [3, 4].

Building Partnerships for Health

1. The Value of Collaboration: Epidemiologists should recognize the expertise and knowledge that communities possess about their own health. Collaborative partnerships between researchers and community members can lead to more relevant, impactful, and sustainable public health interventions.

2. Stakeholder Involvement: Engaging various stakeholders, including community leaders, healthcare providers, educators, and local organizations, can foster a holistic approach to addressing health issues. These stakeholders often have unique perspectives and resources to contribute.

Community-Based Research

1. Community-Centered Research Design: Community-based research actively involves community members in the research process, from defining research questions to data collection and analysis. This approach ensures that the research aligns with the community's needs and priorities.

2. Data Collection in the Community: Conducting surveys, interviews, or data collection activities within the community can improve data quality and community buy-in. It also allows researchers to gather rich contextual information.

Exercise 2: Engaging Your Community in Epidemiological Studies

This exercise encourages readers to explore the principles of community engagement in epidemiological research and practice:

- **Select a Health Issue:** Choose a health issue that is of concern to your community or region. Consider factors, such as disease prevalence, social determinants, and community priorities.
- **Identify Stakeholders:** List the key stakeholders in your community who are relevant to the chosen health issue. This may include community leaders, healthcare providers, local organizations, and affected individuals.
- **Community Engagement Plan:** Develop a community engagement plan outlining how you will involve community members and stakeholders throughout the research process. Consider strategies for building trust, conducting outreach, and involving the community in decision-making.
- **Research Design:** Describe how you will design your epidemiological study to incorporate community perspectives. Will you involve community members in defining research questions, data collection, or analysis? Explain your approach.
- **Data Collection:** Outline your data collection methods and how you plan to conduct research within the community. Consider how you will gather insights, stories, or experiences that may not be captured through traditional epidemiological methods.
- **Community Benefits:** Discuss how your research can benefit the community. Consider how the findings can inform local interventions, policies, or health promotion efforts.
- **Sustainability:** Consider how you will ensure that the engagement of the community continues beyond the research project. Discuss strategies for maintaining partnerships and involving the community in ongoing health initiatives.

By completing Exercise 2, readers can gain a deeper understanding of how to engage their communities in epidemiological studies, fostering collaboration and ensuring that research efforts are rooted in the needs and perspectives of those most affected. This community-centered approach can lead to more effective and sustainable public health outcomes.

CASE STUDIES IN LOCAL EPIDEMIOLOGY

This section highlights the significance of real-life case studies in local epidemiology. By showcasing successful local epidemiological initiatives and discussing the lessons learned, it provides valuable insights for readers [5, 6].

Showcasing Successful Local Epidemiological Initiatives

1. Real-World Examples: Presenting case studies of successful local epidemiological initiatives provides readers with tangible examples of how epidemiological principles can be applied to address local health challenges. These case studies should cover a range of health issues, from infectious diseases to chronic conditions and environmental health concerns.

2. Diverse Settings: Include case studies from various geographical, cultural, and socioeconomic settings. This diversity allows readers to see how epidemiology can be adapted to different contexts and challenges.

3. Collaborative Efforts: Highlight the collaborative nature of these initiatives, emphasizing how multidisciplinary teams, community engagement, and partnerships play a pivotal role in their success.

Lessons Learned and Future Directions

1. Key Takeaways: After presenting each case study, summarize the key lessons learned. These may include insights into effective interventions, challenges faced, and unexpected outcomes.

2. Translating Research into Action: Discuss how the findings and lessons from these case studies are translated into actionable public health strategies, policies, or interventions. Emphasize the impact on local communities.

3. Future Directions: Encourage readers to reflect on how the experiences of these case studies can inform their own epidemiological practice in their local context. Discuss potential future directions for improving local health outcomes.

Exercise 3: Developing Your Local Epidemiological Case Study

This exercise prompts readers to actively engage with local epidemiology through case study development:

- **Choose a Local Health Issue:** Select a health issue or public health challenge that is relevant to your community or region. Consider issues that have received attention or require further investigation.
- **Gather Data:** Collect data and information related to the chosen health issue. This may involve reviewing existing literature, conducting surveys, analyzing local health records, or interviewing community members.
- **Case Study Design:** Design a case study that outlines the background, objectives, methodology, and findings related to the chosen health issue. Include details about the involvement of the community and any partnerships formed.
- **Lessons Learned**: Reflect on the lessons learned from your case study. What insights did you gain, and how can these insights inform local health practices or policies?
- **Future Directions:** Consider the implications of your case study for future public health efforts in your region. How can the findings contribute to better health outcomes, and what steps can be taken to implement these changes?
- **Share Your Case Study**: Share your case study with local stakeholders, public health professionals, or community members to foster discussion and collaboration.

By completing Exercise 3, readers can actively participate in the practice of local epidemiology by developing their case studies. This exercise encourages them to apply epidemiological principles to address local health challenges and contribute to the improvement of community health.

CONCLUSION

In conclusion, Chapter 9 has offered a comprehensive examination of epidemiology in local contexts, encompassing strategies for adaptation, community engagement, and practical application of epidemiological principles. By exploring the unique challenges and characteristics of different regions, readers have gained valuable insights into the importance of tailoring epidemiological methods to address local health needs effectively. Moreover, the chapter underscores the critical role of community engagement in fostering collaboration and trust within local populations, thereby promoting health equity and improving health outcomes. As readers continue to engage with the material presented in the chapter, they will further deepen their understanding of the significance of epidemiology in addressing health disparities and promoting community well-being at the grassroots level.

REFERENCES

[1]   O'Fallon LR, Dearry A. Community-based participatory research as a tool to advance environmental health sciences. Environ Health Perspect 2002; 110(Suppl 2) (Suppl. 2): 155-9.
[http://dx.doi.org/10.1289/ehp.02110s2155] [PMID: 11929724]

[2]   Marmot M, Friel S, Bell R, Houweling TAJ, Taylor S. Closing the gap in a generation: health equity through action on the social determinants of health. Lancet 2008; 372(9650): 1661-9.
[http://dx.doi.org/10.1016/S0140-6736(08)61690-6] [PMID: 18994664]

[3]   Israel BA, Schulz AJ, Parker EA, Becker AB. Review of community-based research: assessing partnership approaches to improve public health. Annu Rev Public Health 1998; 19(1): 173-202.
[http://dx.doi.org/10.1146/annurev.publhealth.19.1.173] [PMID: 9611617]

[4]   Viswanathan M, Ammerman A, Eng E, *et al.* Community-based participatory research: Assessing the evidence. Agency for Healthcare Research and Quality 2004; Vol. 99.

[5]   Scutchfield FD, Keck CW. Principles of public health practice. Cengage Learning 2009.

[6]   Pinto AD, Molnar A, Shankardass K. Have we gone far enough? Monitoring the emergence of community-academic partnerships in Canada's response to the Commission on Social Determinants of Health. Can J Public Health 2016; 107(5-6): e394-6.

SUBJECT INDEX

A

B

C